# Pixiwoo

After both finding careers in the make-up industry, sisters Nic
and Sam joined together to create the Pixiwoo brand. Their highly
successful YouTube makeup channel has over two million
subscribers, with each video generating hundreds of thousands
of views. Sam and Nic are the faces of the globally famous Real
Techniques brush collection. Sam and Nic continue to grow as
top artistic consultants, writing columns for national magazines
and newspapers, appearing on major network television as
beauty experts, and editing their own digital magazine.

# PERFECT EYES

## COMPACT MAKE-UP GUIDE

**EYES • LASHES • BROWS**

# PERFECT
# EYES

## COMPACT MAKE-UP GUIDE

### EYES • LASHES • BROWS

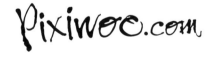

SAM AND NIC CHAPMAN

Published by Blink Publishing
3.25, The Plaza,
535 Kings Road,
Chelsea Harbour,
London, SW10 0SZ

www.blinkpublishing.co.uk

facebook.com/blinkpublishing
twitter.com/blinkpublishing

Perfect Eyes – 978-1-911600-44-2

A CIP catalogue of this book is available from the British Library.

Printed and bound in Lithuania.

1 3 5 7 9 10 8 6 4 2

Text copyright © Samantha Chapman and Nicola Haste/Pixiwoo Limited, 2017
Images © Sam and Nic Chapman, Real Techniques, James Lincoln, Simon Songhurst, Elisabeth Hoff and Shutterstock.
Design by Type & Numbers Creative. www.typeandnumbers.com

Papers used by Blink Publishing are natural, recyclable products made from wood grown in sustainable forests. The manufacturing processes conform to the environmental regulations of the country of origin.

Blink Publishing is an imprint of the Bonnier Publishing Group
www.bonnierpublishing.co.uk

For Mum, without your love and support
none of this would have been possible.

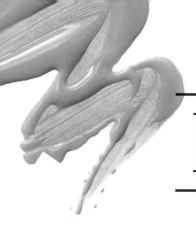
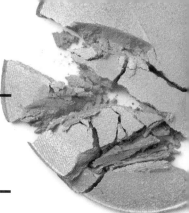

# FACE

APP BY

# Pixiwoo

*THE ULTIMATE* MAKE-UP AND BEAUTY GUIDE ON YOUR SCREEN!

Create the perfect look for every occasion with the Face App by Pixiwoo! The dynamic duo, Sam and Nic Chapman, share their extensive beauty knowledge and make-up expertise with exclusive digital content. From never-before-seen video tutorials, pictures and helpful tips, to special features such as the Selfie Booth, the Face App by Pixiwoo will help you achieve the incredible looks Sam and Nic are known for.

To access all this exclusive content, download the free app from the iTunes App Store or Google Play Store, launch the app and point your device's camera at the pages with the special phone icon (right) on them. Here all of Pixiwoo's advice and special features will come to life on your screen!

*FOR THE ULTIMATE FACE EXPERIENCE DON'T FORGET TO USE YOUR FREE AND UNIQUE PIXIWOO COLOUR WHEEL FOUND IN THE APP'S MAIN MENU*

*The Face App by Pixiwoo requires an Internet connection to be downloaded and can be used on iPhone, iPad or Android devices. For direct links to download the app and further information, visit www.blinkpublishing.co.uk

**SCAN THIS PAGE NOW FOR YOUR FIRST VIDEO!**

# CONTENTS

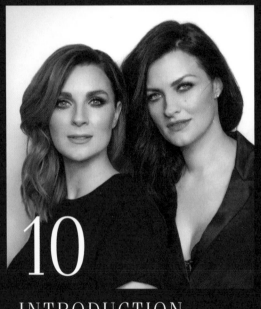

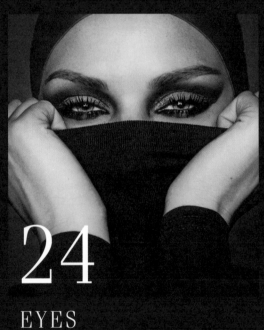

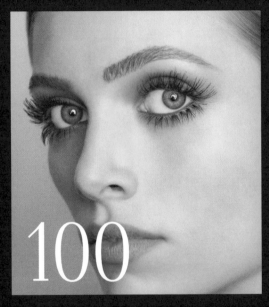

# 100

LASHES

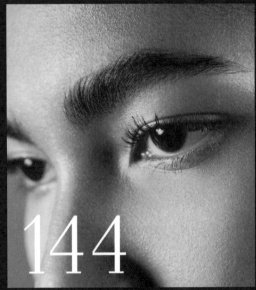

# 144

BROWS

# MEET THE AUTHORS

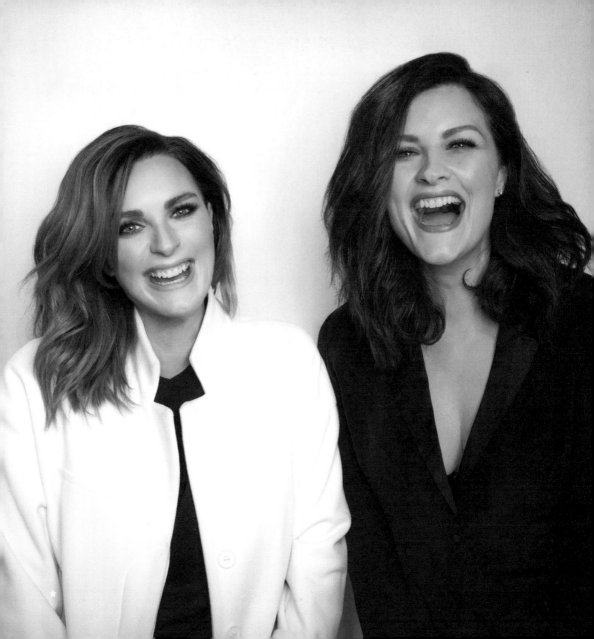

# SAM & NIC

We have been educating women and men of all ages in the art of make-up for over 20 years. We developed Pixiwoo on social media back in 2008.

Pixiwoo was born out of our hard-earned knowledge and passion for make-up and we never imagined it would become our actual career. The success of our channel has enabled us to branch out in many areas.

We have taught hundreds of new make-up artists and we are always inspired by our students' enthusiasm and passion for make-up. We decided to use our knowledge of what people need to learn to produce some easy-to-follow books that break down facial make-up and how to apply it, along with application techniques and our anecdotes and tips.

We wanted to get back to basics and assist beginners or students of the industry and also offer opinions and tips to working make-up artists.

We wanted to also incorporate our social media background and include interactive apps for extra product information, colour theory assistance and brand-new tutorials created especially for you.

You will learn more about us personally, along with our opinions on the best products and also the techniques we normally edit out of our tutorials. You may wonder why we select certain products and tools for our tutorial videos and this book will tell you.

We have loved compiling our knowledge for you and if you are a total make-up beginner and are unsure of where to start then this book will be your companion. If you are just setting out in the industry we will offer you insider tips and advice for your journey.

We hope you enjoy!

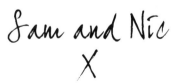

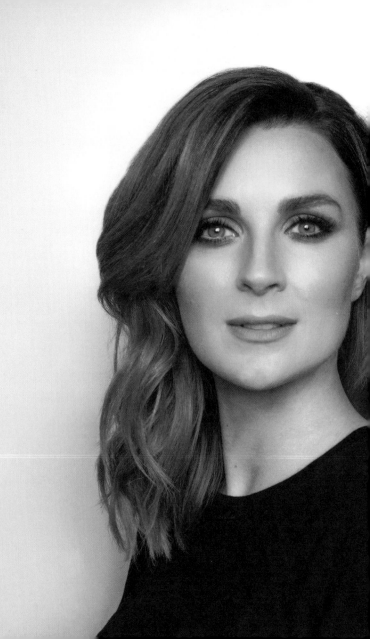

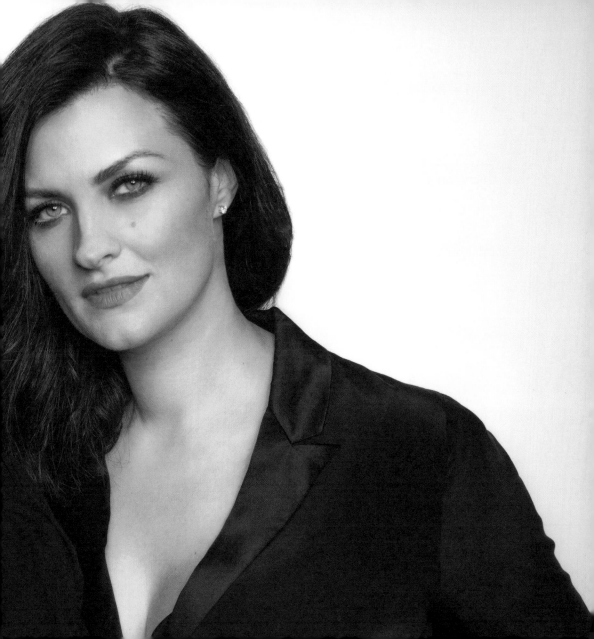

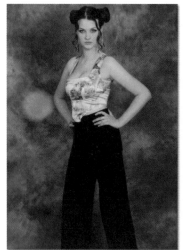

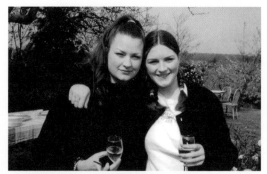

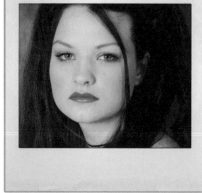

# SAM

I always knew I wanted to do something involving make-up and creativity. As with most siblings, Nic and I squabbled regularly. Nic was the annoying little sister who enjoyed nothing better than trying to wind me up or embarrass me. The only thing that united us was our love of make-up. We loved to watch our mum apply her own make-up and took a great interest in our auntie's career as a make-up artist.

In 1993, after leaving school, I enrolled in a two-year BTEC course in media make-up before moving to London to assist our aunt. I was excited to get away from rural Norfolk and be independent.

I began working on a make-up counter, which gave me confidence with different skin types and tones. I moved to a make-up studio in London where I created suitable looks while working fast.

After two years I began working for MAC in the Carnaby Street Pro Store and later became part of their Pro Team. I travelled extensively to create high-fashion looks for the various fashion weeks and assisted top make-up artists, including Val Garland, Charlotte Tilbury, Sharon Dowsett and Tom Pecheux. Life was pretty hectic but I was really focused on building up my personal portfolio so I would test with other creatives. I also did freelance work including bridal make-up as I was always conscious of having a back-up plan.

In 2003 I got my first agent and was soon booked for magazines and celebrity shoots. I left MAC and worked part-time for Chanel. A year later I had my first daughter, Lily. I continued to work freelance, including doing the make-up for artists at MTV and teaching at a make-up school.

Shortly before the birth of my second daughter, Olivia, I started the Pixiwoo YouTube channel. Nic's childhood nickname was Pixi and my email address then included the word 'Pixiwoo'. I used the name without thinking about how it would become our brand's logo. We like it, though, and there isn't much else out there similar to it.

My first tutorial created a look for a client who wanted a smoky eye. I felt writing the information wouldn't really give her a feel for it – plus I hated to write – so I filmed it instead. The client loved it and more people started to watch and request looks. It started to get really popular and I couldn't manage the workload. By then Nic and I had grown closer and the time we'd spent apart had made us appreciate each other. Nic was always very supportive and was also working in the industry so I asked her if she would like to join me. For two years we worked solidly on the channel, trying to build its popularity. I created tutorials that worked better with my features while Nic's suited her style and look.

The hard work got us noticed and in 2010 Real Techniques approached us. I became Artistic Consultant initially and helped them create a new, different type of make-up brush that performed exceptionally well at an affordable price. The brush range was based on our growing social media success. In 2013, when Nic was able to devote more energy to the brand, we became joint Artistic Consultants. Real Techniques has gone on to become the most popular make-up brush in the UK. It's also now currently the fastest growing make-up brush brand in the US.

We continue to push our brand and never take any of our opportunities for granted. We have worked so hard to build Pixiwoo and we try and take each day as it comes. We still have our fights and have very different ways of approaching situations but we always pull together and make a great team.

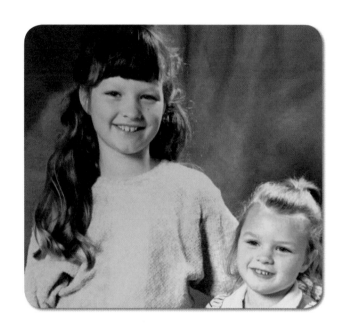

# NICOLA

I was never really academic at school. I loved sports and art but as we grew up in rural Norfolk I was more interested in being outdoors with my friends. I had imagined I would be a nurse as I loved caring for people and this seemed like a natural progression for me.

When I eventually left school I still wasn't quite sure what to do next. Our mum's sister, Maggie, is a successful make-up artist and I loved listening to her talk about her glamorous clients and decided that this might be a fun industry to work in. Sam had already gone on to college to study make-up, and she encouraged me to give it a try. I studied a BTEC National Diploma at college and had a great two years but I still needed extra training and guidance. I don't think you ever really learn until you are in the industry.

I assisted my aunt and also gained valuable work experience at Nicky Clarke and Jo Hansford, both premium hairdressers in London. Based on my good work ethic they both offered me a job, but I was focused on make-up.

I returned to Norfolk and landed a job for Estée Lauder working on the counter and gradually worked my way up to counter manager. I heard that there was a MAC store coming to Norwich and working for a sister brand helped me to get an interview.

I was so excited and I can still remember the make-up I wore. A combination of So There Jade and Minted eyeliner, a vibrant green mascara called Boston Fern and a baby pink lipstick called Snob. It was a winning combination and I became an assistant manager.

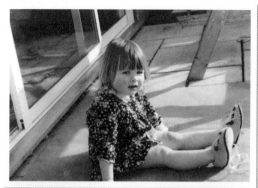

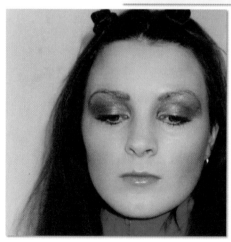

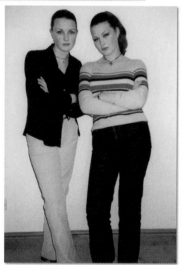

I remained in this position for four years and made some great friends before becoming a supervisor at the MAC Pro Store in Carnaby Street, London, for three years. I would often freelance in the evenings – bridal work, drag make-up and editorial work. Then I joined Illamasqua in Selfridges.

In 2008 Sam told me that she had started recording make-up tutorials on YouTube and had begun to get lots of requests for looks. She asked if I wanted to help create some tutorials. Sam never really had a massive plan but we decided to create fun and informative content.

I really enjoyed helping her but it was hard working full-time and freelancing too. I decided that I would return home to Norfolk and give this YouTube thing a go! I knew I could always fall back on bridal make-up work. We started creating looks for the channel and at the weekend we worked together as bridal make-up artists to earn some money. This was the first time in years we had been in each other's presence regularly but the time apart had drawn us closer.

I soon met my husband, Ian, and I knew that Norfolk was where I wanted to be so Sam and I focused really hard on the Pixiwoo channel. In 2010 we were approached by Real Techniques to help create a new type of make-up brush. Sadly I had two miscarriages and just needed to focus on myself. I just helped behind the scenes at Real Techniques. Fortunately, Ian and I went on to have two beautiful children, Harry and Edie. I then joined the Real Techniques team with Sam as an Artistic Consultant while creating weekly tutorials for Pixiwoo.

We never like to plan too far ahead and take each day as it comes. We know each other's strengths and also when the other is struggling. Every week brings a new challenge but we deal with it together.

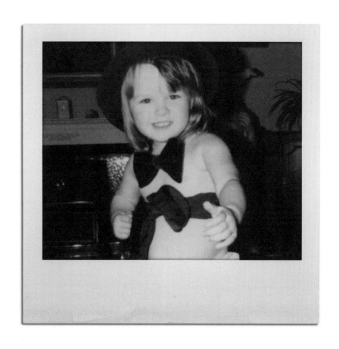

# EYES

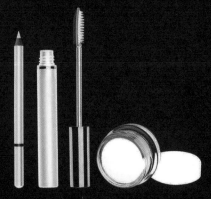

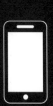

*"Beauty is something you feel
inside and it reflects in your eyes.
It's not physical."*

———————————— *Sophia Loren*

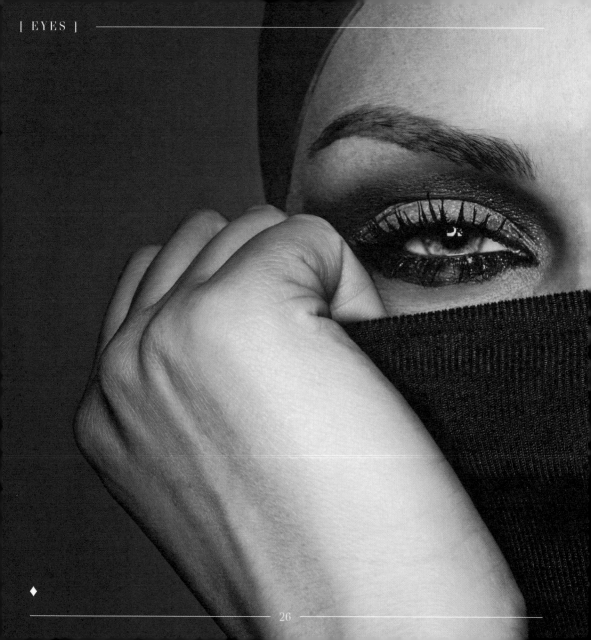

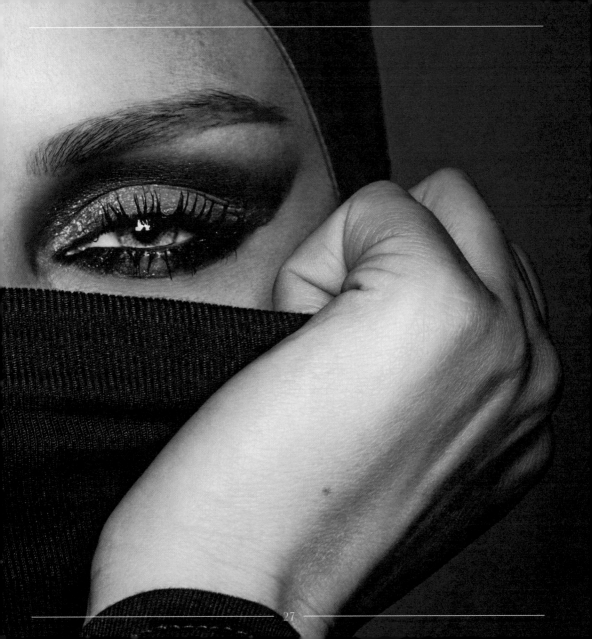

YOU MAY HAVE *ONE EYE* WHICH IS *A DIFFERENT SIZE* OR *SHAPE* FROM *THE OTHER* SO *IT'S IMPORTANT* TO IDENTIFY *YOUR SHAPE* SO THAT YOU CAN *BEST APPLY* PRODUCT.

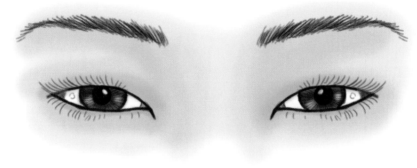

## MONOLID

'Mono' translates as 'one' and a monolid is one lid. It doesn't have a socket line or a crease. When looked at in profile the lid appears flat from the eyebrow down to the lash line. It can sometimes appear a little puffy.

You will know if you have a monolid when you look directly into a mirror because you will see flat skin rather than a crease.

Find your natural eye crease or socket line by locating the socket bone right above your eyeball. The crease falls below that bony area.
You can create a crease by using a dark eyeshadow, but you need to be quite

skilled at make-up application. It looks great from a distance but close up it can be quite obviously fake. A false crease sits just above the eye and needs to be blended well. Place the crease in exactly the same position on the opposite eye.

Working on make-up counters we encountered women who used eyelid tape on their monolids. These slim slithers of sticky tape, popular in the Far East, adhere to the lid and are pushed into the orbit of the eye to create a socket. The tape is usually transparent, although this can sometimes make it tricky to apply colour over the top. They can be purchased in eyeshadow colours or in black to help them blend in when wearing full eye make-up.

Apply your eyeshadow in a block across the lash line and blend the colour upwards – darker at the lash line and lighter as it blends towards the brow. Liquid or gel liner at the lash line works well at giving definition.

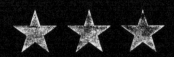

*Tip – Monolid eyelashes
can be very short or dead straight,
so apply false lashes to
dramatically enhance the eyes.*

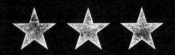

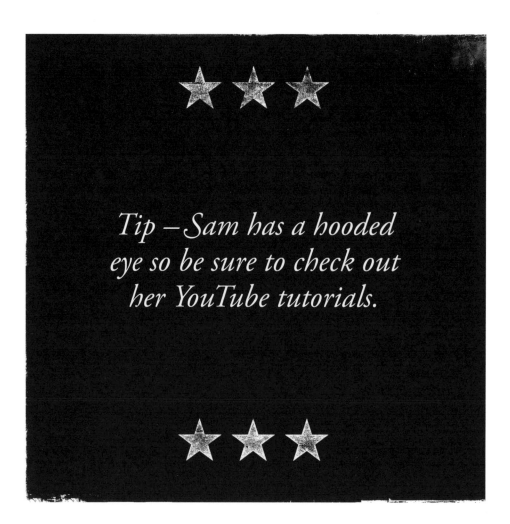

*Tip — Sam has a hooded eye so be sure to check out her YouTube tutorials.*

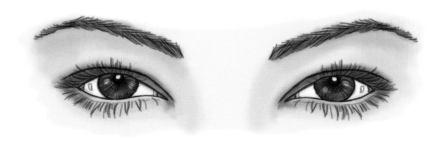

## HOODED EYES

Some people are born with a hooded eyelid and some develop one as they age. Either way, the upper lid falls over your natural crease. It can resemble a monolid by hiding the crease underneath the upper lid.

To see where to apply colour in your natural crease, hold a mirror low and look down into it. Any colour applied to the socket will be covered by the hooded lid.

Apply eyeshadow in the same way as you would for a monolid, with the strongest amount of colour at the lash line, blending upwards in a block. The colour should run in a gradient from dark through to light. You may need to take your eyeshadow higher towards the brow. Also try winging the eyeshadow out at the edges of the eye. This creates a feline effect and gives the eye an almond shape. Corner eyelashes at the outer edge of the eye will enhance this type of shadow application.

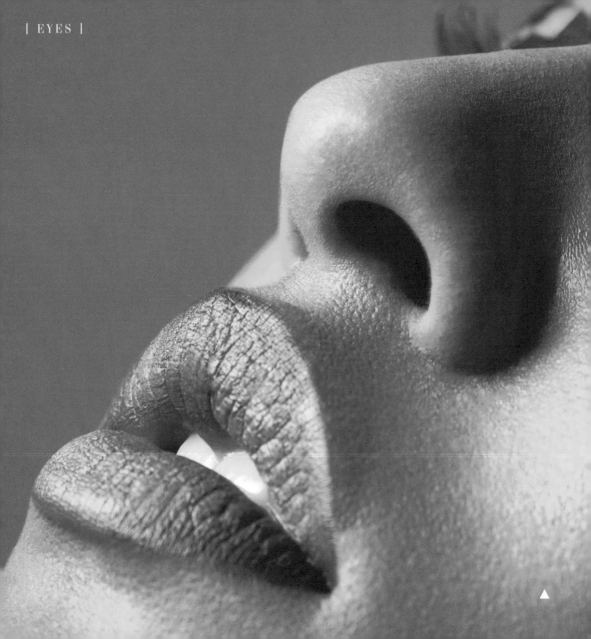

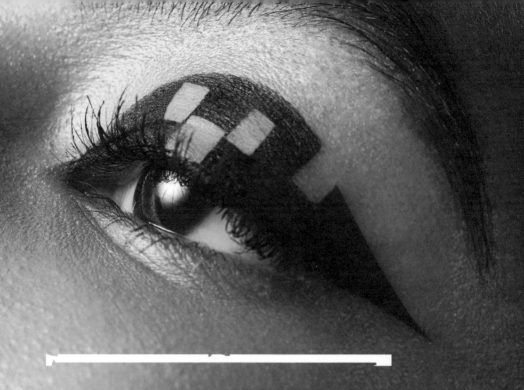

THE *EYES* ARE
THE *FIRST FEATURE*
WE *NOTICE.*

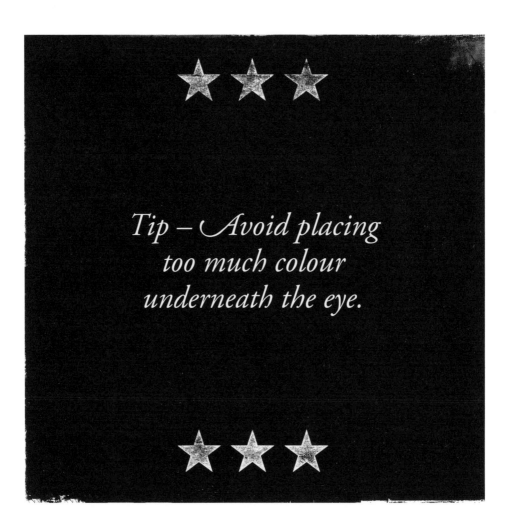

*Tip – Avoid placing
too much colour
underneath the eye.*

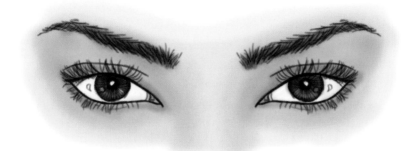

We love this shape. It's the classic almond shape and looks very youthful. Imagine there is a line running horizontally through the centre of your pupil as you look straight in a mirror. The outer corners of an upturned eye will sit higher than the imaginary line.

To balance upturned corners, keep the eyeshadow at the outer edge of the eyelid darker and blend it softly around and under the eye. Apply eyeshadow or a pencil liner along the corner of the bottom lashes. This will make the lower lash line appear even and lowered.

Use a kohl or pencil liner on the waterline of the eye, the fleshy part of the inner lower lash line, from where your lower eye lashes project. Keep the kohl to the outer edge. Apply more mascara to the bottom lashes than the top to draw attention away from the upturned corner.

CURLING THE *UPPER LASHES* AND APPLYING *CORNER FALSE LASHES* WILL *ENHANCE* AND *LIFT* THE *OUTER EDGE*.

## DOWNTURNED EYES

Imagine a line running horizontally through the pupil. If the outer edge of the eye sits below that line then the eyes are downturned. They can seem slightly sad.

Your eyes can be lifted at the edges if you keep your darkest eyeshadow on the upper lid and blend upwards towards the corner of the brow. You can also use pencil or liquid liner along the upper lash line and create a winged flick, angled upwards.

Curling the upper lashes and applying corner false lashes will enhance and lift the outer edge.

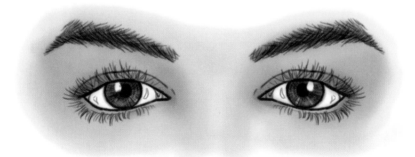

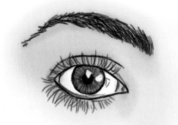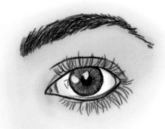

### ROUND EYES

You can often see the whites of round eyes around the iris and you can combat this by creating a more elongated shape. At the most rounded area of the upper eyelid, keep the darkest eyeshadow close to the lash line and blend the eyeshadow straight across towards the outer edge.

Start eyeliner at the outer corner of the iris and wing it out in a straight line rather than following the shape of the eye. Mirror the eyeshadow shape under the eye, sweeping it along in a straight line towards the outer edge.

Don't curl your eyelashes as this will enhance the centre of the eye. Apply less mascara to the middle section of the eye and give the inner and outer corner lashes a good coat of mascara. Very short, individual lashes applied to the inner and outer corner of the eye can help.

Correcting small eyes is more about eyeshadow colour. Choose lighter colours that have a light reflective finish. Using a wash of a light-coloured, reflective eyeshadow over the lid will open the eyes. Keep darker eyeshadow to the outer edge and socket line of the eyes, creating an inverted 'C' shape at the edge. Don't apply your eyeshadow in a block all the way along the eyelid.

Avoid eyeshadow under the lower lashes. Blend a soft liner across the upper lash line and wing it out softly. Use a flesh-coloured or off-white eye pencil in the waterline of the lower eye. This will instantly brighten and whiten the eye. Give the lashes a good curl and apply lashings of mascara to both top and bottom lashes.

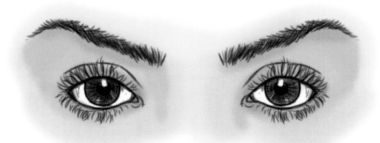

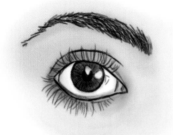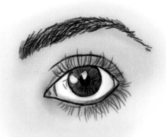

## PROTRUDING EYES

You will never totally be able to make your protruding eye appear flat. The natural shape of your eye will always be there. But you can help by avoiding overly shimmery products or light-reflecting colours that project light and make the eyes more prominent.

Matte eyeshadow (especially darker shades) is your best weapon. Apply your shadow just as you would for round eyes, using an eye kohl in any dark shade to the waterline of the eye from the inner corner across to the outer corner.

If you are confident, apply the same pencil to the waterline of the upper eyelid also. By coating the upper and lower waterlines of the eye you will downplay the projection.

## CLOSE-SET EYES

Evenly spaced eyes, in theory, would allow another eye to fit between them. If not, they are close-set, when the inner corners of each eye appear to be very close to the side of the nose, with more space at the outer corner.

Use light-coloured eyeshadow on the inner corner and blend a darker colour at the outer, drawing the outer edge more widely. You can use liner, beginning at the start of the iris of the eye and winging out to make your desired shape. Keep your mascara to the outer edge and don't apply any to the fine lashes on the inner corner.

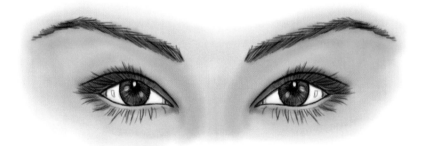

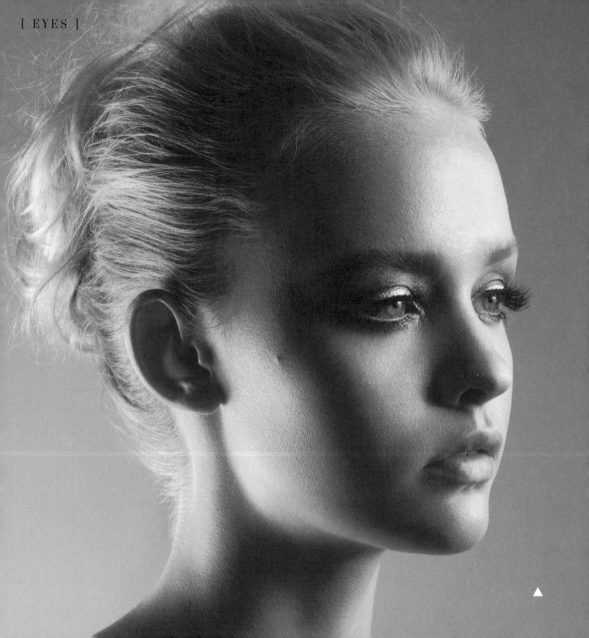

## WIDE-SET EYES

If another eye could easily fit between your eyes you can draw the eyes together. Apply eyeshadow in a block all over the eyelid and use a little bronzer through the inner corner and inner socket of your eye. This will create a natural-looking shadow on the inside of the eye.

Line the inner corners of your waterline with a kohl to give the illusion of the eyes sitting closer together. Focus your mascara on the inner, fine lashes with a sheer application to the outer edge.

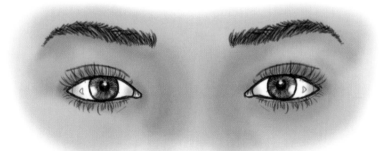

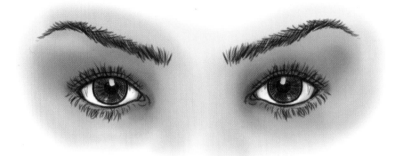

## DEEP-SET EYES

You will know if you have deep-set eyes because your brow bone protrudes further than your eyeball. Strong, high cheekbones may accentuate this.

Bring the eyes forward with light eyeshadow shades. Shimmer or satin-finish eyeshadows will also help achieve a brighter, more open eyelid.

Curling the lashes and using tons of mascara draw the eyes forward. Coloured mascara also works really well, drawing attention to the eyes and brightening the area. Be sure to also keep your brow shape in check, tweezing low-lying hairs to open up the eye area.

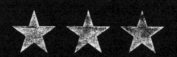

*Tip – You can use an
eyeshadow that's a few
shades darker than your
natural skin tone.*

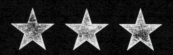

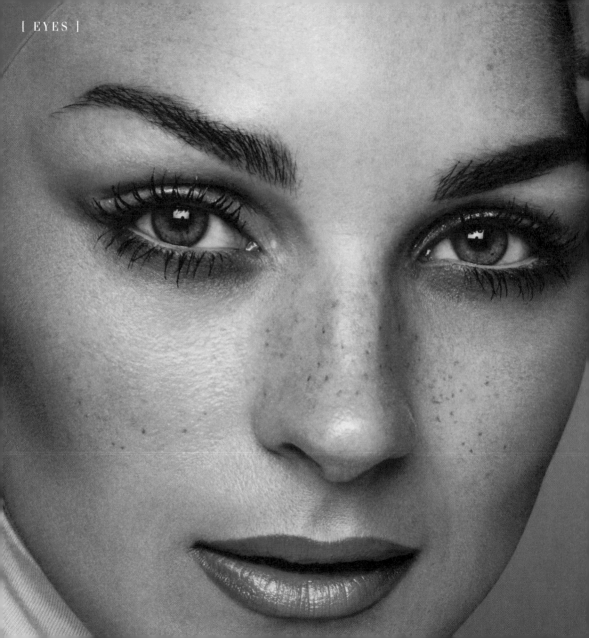

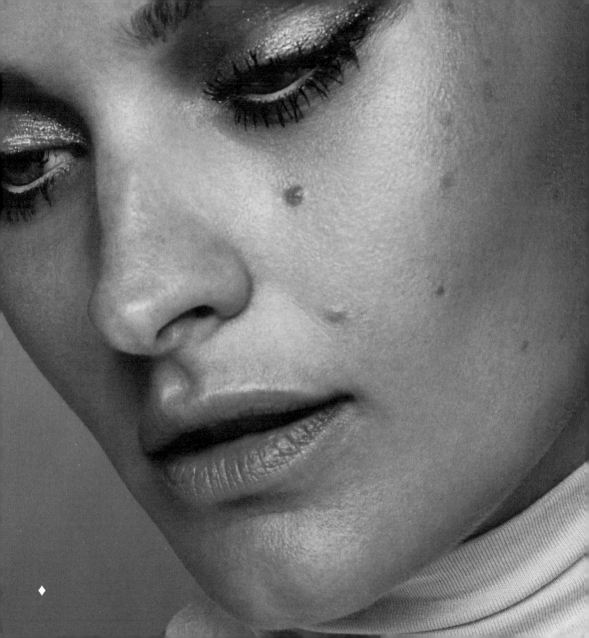

## EYE MAKE-UP FOR GLASSES AND CONTACT LENS WEARERS

Spectacle wearers always ask us how to use make-up to enhance their eyes and just because you wear glasses doesn't mean you have to compromise on your make-up. Application can be the hardest part – you might not be able to see what you're doing without them but you can't put it on wearing them!

Your eyes can get a little lost behind frames. Rimless glasses are great unless you need frames to support stronger prescription lenses, when you can try a lighter-coloured, ombré or thinner frame. Frames upturned in an almond shape show more of the sides of the eyes.

You can guide application with a lighted magnifying mirror on a stand, leaving your hands free to support your eyelid and apply colour. Specialist make-up eyeglasses work really well although they do look a little crazy. Each magnified lens is on a hinge and while one is flipped up you can see through the other.

Apply your eye make-up as we recommend, but perhaps try a brighter shade or go a little darker to make it stand out. Eyeliner gives the eyes definition if you don't want to wear eyeshadow. A thin application of liquid liner to the upper lashes or soft kohl pencil blended around and under the eye enhances the shape and adds definition.

Long, luscious lashes can hit glasses and bend back or feel uncomfortable when you wear mascara. Try eyelash tinting. You can still have the dark lashes without the curl.

If you wear contact lenses, remember that eyeshadow powders with glitter or a granular texture may drop down into the eye and cause irritation. Avoid them or apply your make-up before you put in your lenses and always carry a spare pair.

Some mascaras that provide volume may contain tiny nylon fibres that cling to the lashes to enhance their thickness and length. These fibres inevitably drop and cling to contact lenses and these mascaras are best avoided. You can spot them by the tiny, hair-like pieces they leave on the wand.

Stick to the use-by date on all products. Ageing make-up becomes dry, flaky and harbours bacteria that can get onto the lens and cause pretty nasty eye infections.

THE *TRICK WITH EYE PRIMER* IS TO *APPLY A SMALL* AMOUNT, *BUFFED OVER* THE *EYELID* WITH A *FLUFFY BRUSH*.

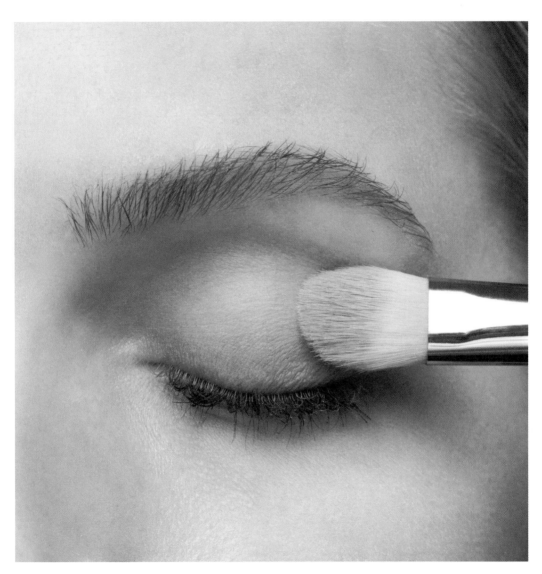

## EYE PRIMER

Primers can help with longevity and if you have oily eyelids or are in a humid country. They will contain talc that helps to absorb oil from the lid and colour to stay in place.

Primers can be applied all over the eyelid and up to the brow, providing a barrier between the skin and any cosmetic product. They help to prevent creasing and movement of your eyeshadow and aid in its blending. To combat discolouration or dullness on the lid, look for primers tinted in a peach tone or those containing light-reflective pigments.

Universal eye primers can be colourless or coloured for a specific tone. Very deep skin tones require a peach or golden tint. The trick with eye primer is to apply a small amount, buffed over the eyelid with a fluffy brush. A sheer veil absorbs oil and dries quickly so you can instantly apply eyeshadow without slipping on the lid and causing a crease.

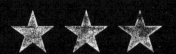

*Tip – Assess your eyelids throughout the day – you may not even need a primer.*

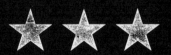

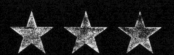

*Tip – The best way to apply
a cream eyeshadow is using
a synthetic brush, which doesn't
absorb the product.*

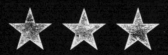

## CREAM EYESHADOW

We adore cream eyeshadows. They are a super-easy texture to work with, are very forgiving of mistakes and work well with powder eyeshadow to give more vibrancy.

Creams usually come in a pot or in a twist-up lipstick-style applicator. Screw the lid on tightly otherwise the cream dries and shrinks.

Cream eyeshadow can be worn on its own as a sheer wash over the eye or you can blend multiple cream colours, remembering they will merge rather than settling on the skin separately as powders do.

Some creams dry on the skin, which is great for longevity, but blend quickly to avoid a patchy finish.

Cream eyeshadows make a fantastic base for your powder eyeshadow. We actually prefer to use them as a base instead of a primer, but stick with a primer if you have oily eyelids. Cream eyeshadow evens out the eyelid and helps any powder eyeshadow you apply to adhere and appear more vibrant and bold.

Create a unique colour by applying a vibrant-coloured cream eyeshadow underneath a contrasting powder eyeshadow. Powder is a safer option on a mature lid, as creams sink into creases and enhance the skin texture over fine lines. You can use a primer to combat this but the cream usually always settles.

## POWDER EYESHADOW

Powder eyeshadows are widely used as eyeshadow texture. They are either pressed into a pot or in a palette alongside complementary shades.

Powder eyeshadows can be hit or miss. Some are formulated well, have good-quality ingredients and are carefully pressed into the compact. Cheaper ingredients may be crumbly, smash easily in the palette and also cause 'fall-out' or 'drop-down', when powder particles drop onto the cheek (and carpet!) in application.

Some colour pigments used in eyeshadow drop more than others. In our experience, black, purple and blue powder eyeshadows are the worst offenders.

Powder eyeshadows can be divided into many categories depending on the finish and each brand has its own terminology.

## MATTE FINISH

This texture has zero shine or shimmer. It is a flat, one-dimensional colour and can be tricky to work with as it has a much dryer formula. Matte shades are notoriously hard to blend and darker matte shades can go patchy.

Matte textures create a beautiful, intense, smoky eye and are also great to use as a contour colour through the socket of the eye. They mimic the skin's natural texture. They can also be used as an eyeliner along the lash line for a softer look. On a mature eye, they sit particularly nicely as a liner because they don't move or crease.

## PEARL FINISH

This is a two-tone finish that reflects differently depending on the light. They usually blend easily and have a good pay-off, by which we mean a strongly pigmented colour.

This finish works well over a cream eyeshadow, taking on the colour and texture of the cream underneath and giving off a unique colour – think of the effect of water and oil mixing on the roadside.

## SATIN

This resembles the finish of satin fabric. It has a natural, even sheen with no glitter or frosting. Generally, these finishes blend really well and complement all skin types and ages.

## FROSTED

Frosted shadows are infused with glitter particles. Depending on the quality, you will get a shimmering base colour that reflects the light. However, it can be difficult to get an even blend because of the sporadic glitter and particles can also drop down into the eye. It's not great for contact lens wearers and can be a problem on mature skin.

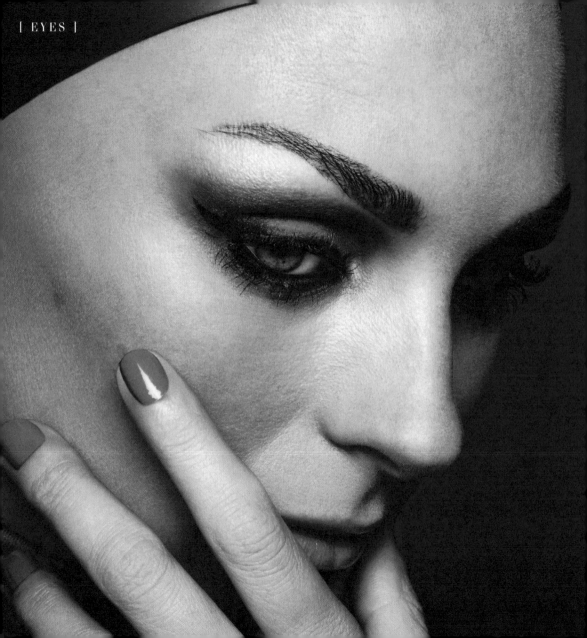

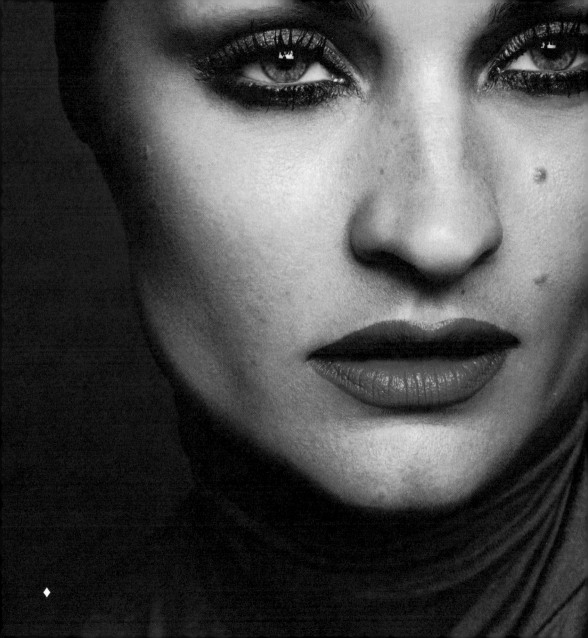

EYESHADOW *POWDERS* COME IN A *LOOSE FORM* SO THAT THEY *CAN BE MIXED* WITH *OTHER PRODUCTS* AND USED ON *OTHER AREAS*.

## VELVET

This can have a similar finish as a satin finish, but it feels more luxurious. It sometimes has a soft light-reflective finish and can be good for blending and layering with other textures.

## LOOSE-POWDER EYESHADOW

Eyeshadow powders come in a loose form so that they can be mixed with other products and used on other areas. They are often referred to as pigments by some brands. You can apply onto a clean eyelid, but they adhere better with a cream eyeshadow underneath.

Use as an eyeshadow with a firm brush, patting the colour into the eyelid. Don't blend it over with a fluffy brush which will cause the product to drop down. Loose-powder eyeshadows can also be used as blushers, but sparingly, as they are often strongly pigmented.

Light-coloured loose-powder eyeshadows such as bronze or silver can be mixed with face or body moisturiser to give skin a soft radiance. Body painters mix loose powder colours to create new, unique shades. Another fun use for them is to add colour to a clear mascara.

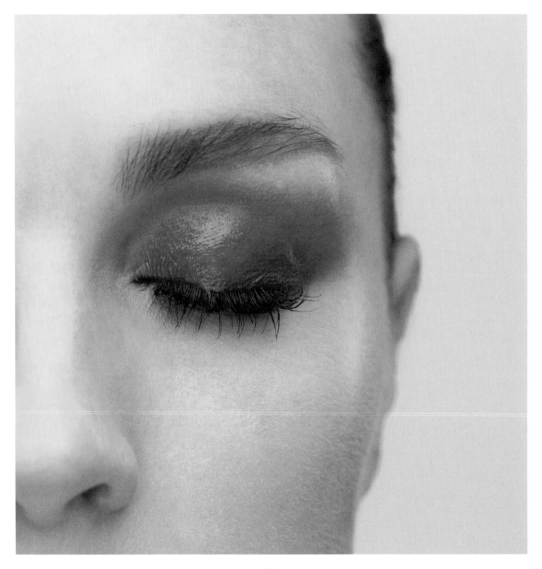

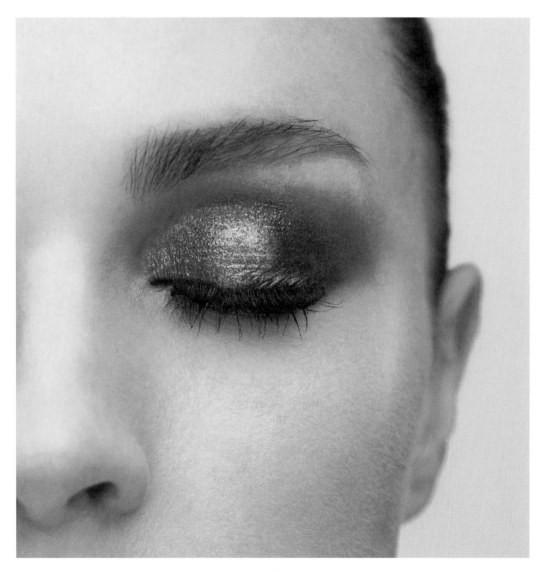

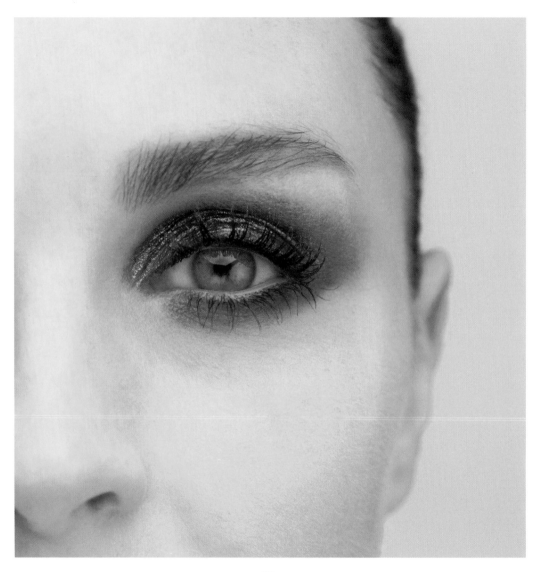

## GLITTER PIGMENTS

Like magpies, we are attracted to our little pots of loose glitter particles. Brands recommend that these are only used on the face and body – covering themselves in case you get glitter in your eye and scratch your retina! We use glitter around our eyes all the time without problems but it's down to you to decide if you want to take the (very minimal) risk.

The larger the pieces of glitter, the more likely they are to drop into the eye. Tiny, fine glitter particles won't really cause any more irritation than a frosted eyeshadow.

First coat the lid with cream eyeshadow or eye gel. Some brands sell mixing medium, a creamy film with the texture of petroleum jelly.

Using a firm brush, press the glitter onto the lid. Bits of glitter will drop down so apply your base afterwards, having first used a facial wet wipe to clear up.

Make-up artists working in studios remember that chunky shards of glitter don't photograph well. Light bounces off and reflects as a dull, grey square. Fine glitter, however, looks beautiful in the flesh and on camera, reflecting light to create a wash of shimmering colour.

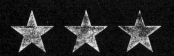

*Tip – Be extra cautious
if you have sensitive eyes
or wear contact lenses.*

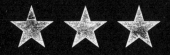

## EYE COLOUR THEORY

There are no strict rules if you feel confident with contrasting colours or experimenting. The rest of us may find it useful to follow basic colour theory guidelines.

## BROWN EYES

You are so lucky. Pretty much anything will go with your brown eyes, but be careful to check them, as eyes almost always contain a few flecks or tints of other colours.

Using brown colours, keep a warm, chocolate tone with a red pigment. This will enhance the richness of your eyes and create a beautiful, smoky effect.

Enhance light brown eyes with green or yellow flecks by wearing a plum- or purple-based eyeshadow. Warm taupes and any golds, from pale yellow through to warm bronzes, will also work. Olive greens can look fab with brown eyes, and navy or bright cobalt blue create a striking contrast.

## BLUE EYES

Most colours will go with blue but be careful of making them appear red or sore-looking. Avoid any shades of frosty pink or red-based browns. Orange and gold will make your blue eyes look insanely bright. Orange pigment next to blue creates a vibrant shade (think of how the sun makes the sea into a dazzling

*ORANGE* AND *GOLD* WILL *MAKE YOUR BLUE EYES* LOOK *INSANELY BRIGHT*.

turquoise) and gold- and terracotta-toned browns work in the same way. If you wish, you can wear blue on a blue eye but a deeper shade of blue works better. Navy or indigo work especially well.

## GREEN EYES

Slate grey and black complement a green eye beautifully, as do silver and soft olive green. Apply any shade of purple to make a green eye colour pop, from lilac through to a regal purple and plum to blackberry. Cool-toned taupe and forest green will also look stunning.

## GREY EYES

Black, smoky colours look great for the evening and any blue, from cornflower through to midnight blue, should work well. Warm-toned purples will make the eyes appear slightly more green or grey and neutral, soft browns sit nicely for a daytime look.

## HAZEL EYES

Being a mix of brown and green you can wear the colours we have recommended for both eye colours. If your eyes have a lot of yellow tones in them use a metallic bronze.

# DARK *SMOKY EYESHADOW* CAN REALLY *INTENSIFY LIGHT* EYES AND *FRAME* DARK EYES.

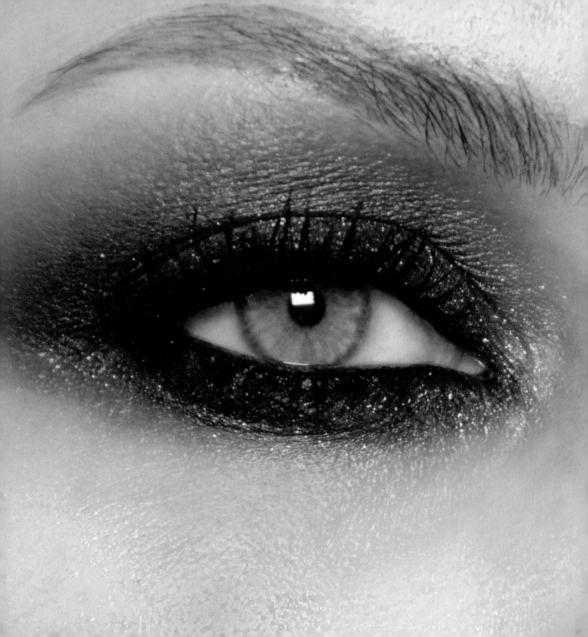

## HOW TO BLEND EYESHADOW

Most importantly, you need to ensure you have the best tools for the job. If you are working with two or more eyeshadow products, you will need at least four clean brushes.

Ensure you have a fluffy blending brush to apply your base colour. This should be synthetic if you are using a cream base or natural hair if you are using a powder. You will also need at least two flat brushes to apply colour and another clean blending brush to buff the shades into each other.

Don't even attempt to use those small sponge applicators that are sold in eyeshadow palettes. They are hard to blend with, drag the delicate skin around the eye and are impossible to clean.

If using dark colours, we find it easier to complete our eye make-up before our foundation. Simply clean the drop-down with a facial wipe before you begin your base.

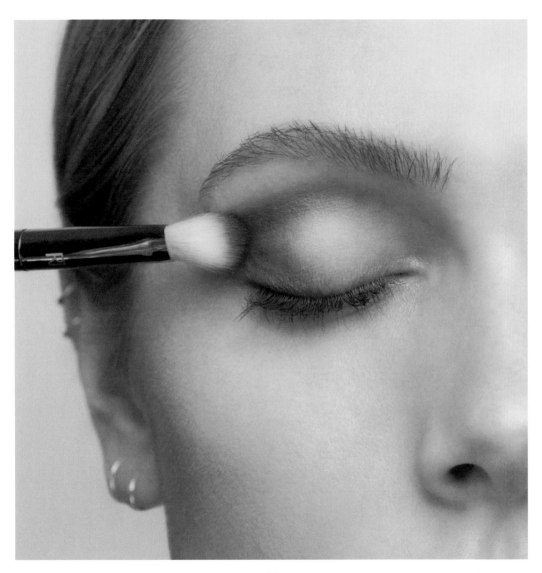

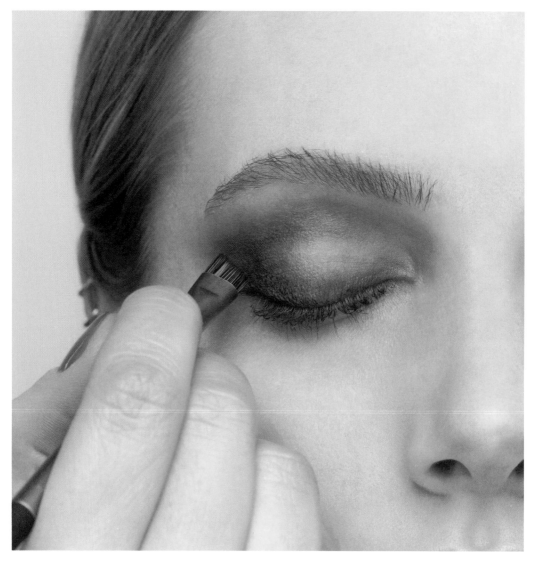

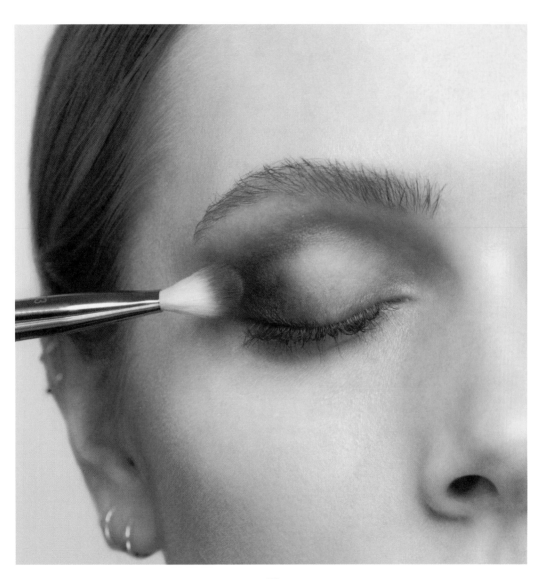

Here is a step-by-step guide for well-blended eyeshadow:

## 1

Use a colour similar to your own skin colour all over the eyelid. This will even your skin tone and create a base for the other colours. It also helps longevity. Cream base gives a more vibrant result.

## 2

Depending on the shape you are creating, apply your next colour with a firm, flat brush all over the moveable part of the lid up to the socket or just apply it at the outer edge and through the socket of the eye in an inverted 'C', depending on your eye shape.

## 3

Using a fluffy brush, blend this colour into the skin. You can apply more of the colour with a flat brush if needed but be sure to blend between each layer.

## 4

We like to dust our bronzer or blusher shade over the socket line of the eye. This blends edges, creates a natural contour and ties the whole look together. Use a soft, fluffy brush.

## 5

Use a flat brush to add highlight colours to the inner corner of the eye or under the brow bone.

## 6

Use a smaller flat brush to take the eyeshadow under the eye, under the lower lashes and blend well.

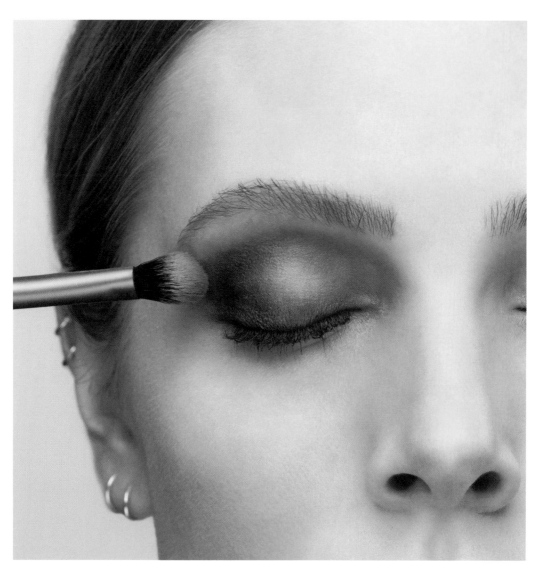

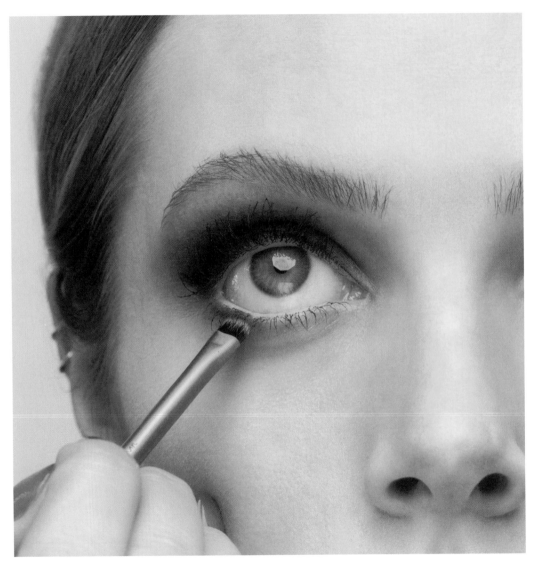

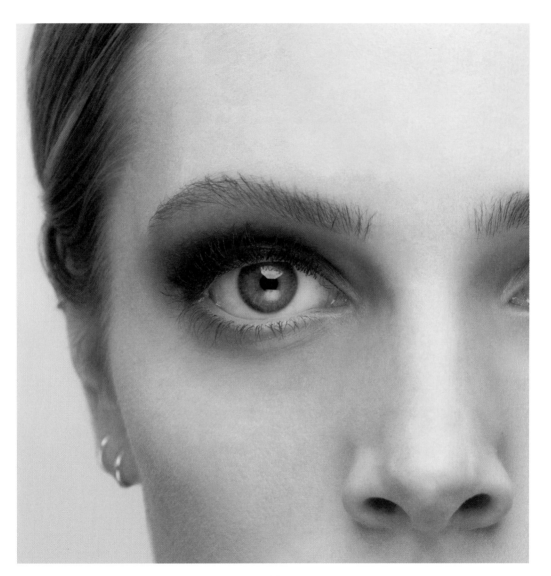

*SIMPLE EYELINER CAN ADD DEFINITION, CREATE SHAPE OR HELP WITH ITS CORRECTION AND TURN A DAY LOOK INTO AN EVENING LOOK.*

# [ EYELINERS ]

## PENCIL LINERS

A pencil will give a defined, fine line with a firm application, but remember to sharpen it with a cosmetic pencil sharpener. These are angled precisely to fit and usually contain a fine surgical blade to give an ultra-fine point.

Pencils don't blend as well as an eye kohl. Great for people who don't like a smudgy, blended finish and good for a watery eye as the line holds its shape.

They last well in the waterline of the eye, but you don't want any sharp, scratchy points near your eyeball so run the pencil over the back of your hand first to soften that point.

## KOHL PENCILS

Much softer than a pencil. Usually contains beeswax to help soften the product and to assist colour transfer onto the skin.

Kohls are the best option for a smudgy, soft line that blends easily and great to use in place of a cream eyeshadow. Apply as a base all over the eyelid and blend fast as they tend to dry quicker than a cream, going patchy and making it hard for you to then blend in a powder. You can also use these in the waterline of the eye but they move and wear away faster than a pencil.

## FLESH-TONE PENCILS

'Flesh tone' is such a horrid name but it's the best way to describe these pencils coloured in natural skin tone shades. They are designed to be worn in the waterline of the eye, lightening its pink or red tone and creating a brighter, healthy-looking eye that looks more natural and modern than a white pencil. Light, pastel-toned liners add a flash of colour.

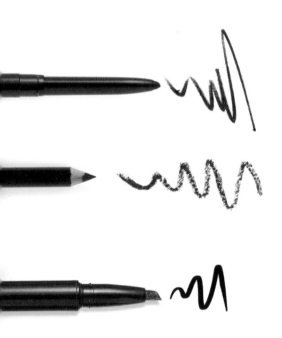

## LIQUID LINERS

Liquid liner is notoriously hard to apply, or at least to get even on both eyes! There are different textures of liquid liner available though and some are easier to use than others.

## FELT-TIP PEN-STYLE LINERS

These usually have a soft, flexible tip that applies easily. The texture is not too wet so you can build a precise shape and correct mistakes, but they dry out after three months and faster if you don't replace the cap firmly.

## INKPOT-STYLE LINERS

The pots have a fine, firm application wand in the lid but the product is very wet and hard to control and better used by professionals.

The firm point creates delicate, intricate designs but drying takes longer and if you have hooded or deep-set eyes, liners will annoyingly transfer to the skin.

## GEL LINERS

Our favourite and the easiest for beginners to use, although they are not sold with a brush. The gel texture is thick and easy to control. A small amount makes a strong impact and the colour pay-off is good.

Apply with a fine or angled liner brush. Dip in the brush, wipe off the excess and apply to the lash line. Begin with a light covering and build up the gel to increase depth and colour.

## CAKE LINERS

These old-fashioned liners – similar to eye-shadow but with a waxier texture – are unhygienic and no longer widely used. They dry out quickly, crack and crumble apart. You have to dampen your brush or spritz a little water into the product before applying. They do remain popular in the theatre for creating strong, graphic looks that last under strong lighting.

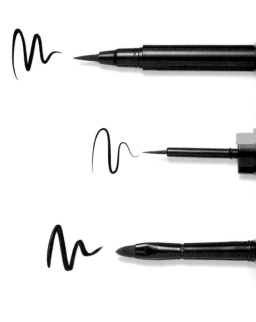

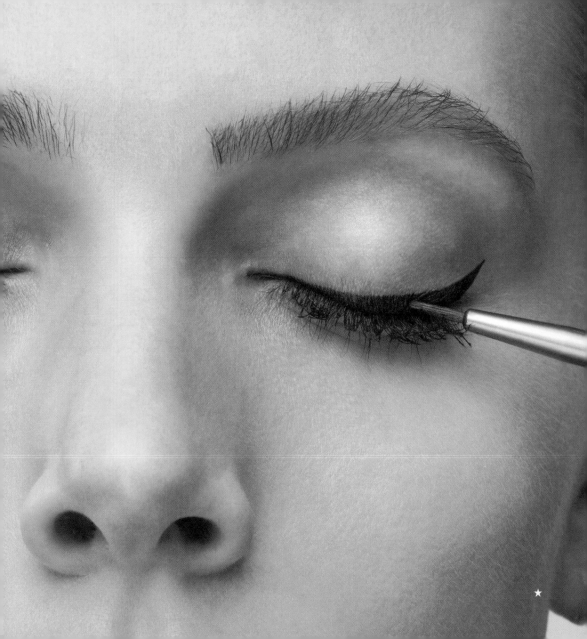

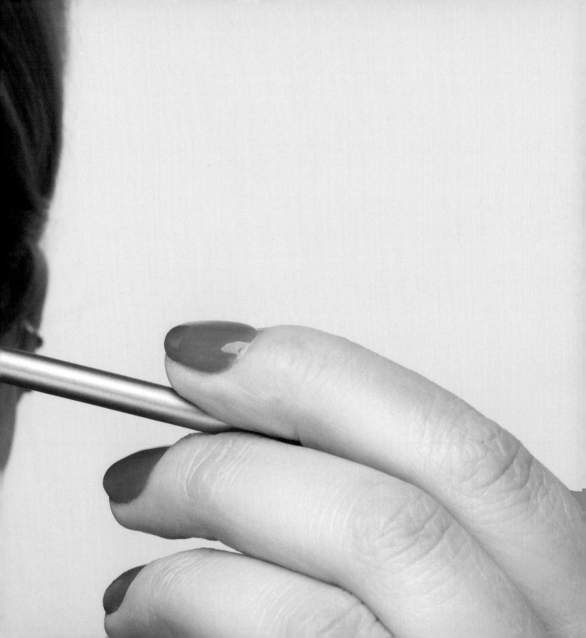

## HOW TO APPLY LIQUID LINER

We touched on this in the eye-shape section and here is a general guide
to follow for a basic liner shape:

# 1

Never close your eye while you apply or you may find the tail of your
liner flick goes off at a weird angle. Skin is looser when the eye is open
and its creases cut through the applied liner.

# 2

We like to have both an angled brush and a fine liner brush ready.
Make sure they are clean, dry and neat.

# 3

Keep a few cotton buds saturated with eye make-up remover
at hand to touch up or correct mistakes.

# 4

Position your mirror – not a hand-held – directly in front of you.

# 5

Using your brush or liner application wand, apply the flick of your liner at the outer edge of the eye. Apply a faint line, following the line of your bottom lash line around to the edge of your eye. You can build up and darken this later.

# 6

Repeat for the second eye.

# 7

Check your flicks. If they are uneven, remove and reapply. Better now than having to remove your whole liner later.

# 8

You can now close one eye and, starting from the inner corner, paint on your liner close to the lashes. With the flicks in place, you can see where to join up.

# 9

You should have a natural line that you can build on, darken and thicken.

You may have seen us talking about tight lining the eye. This means filling in the upper waterline that sits between your eye and the roots of your upper lashes. After applying make-up and liner you can sometimes still see pink skin under your lashes and by filling this in you will complete a much darker, smokier look.

Do this before you apply mascara. Use a soft kohl pencil. Look down into a mirror, gently pull your lid up and quickly fill in the fleshy area. Close your eye and apply a kohl liner along the lash line.

Use tape to create an extreme, winged-out liner if you don't have a steady hand. Tape helps to create unique eyeshadow shapes with a defined, sharp edge.

We recommend micro-pore tape, a latex-free, hypoallergenic paper tape originally designed to hold bandages in place and available online or from chemists. It's made of paper and you can tear it to the length required. You can apply your eyeshadow or liner over the straight edge to make a sharp line.

# PRACTISE, PRACTISE, PRACTISE. *THAT* IS THE *KEY* TO *SUCCESS*.

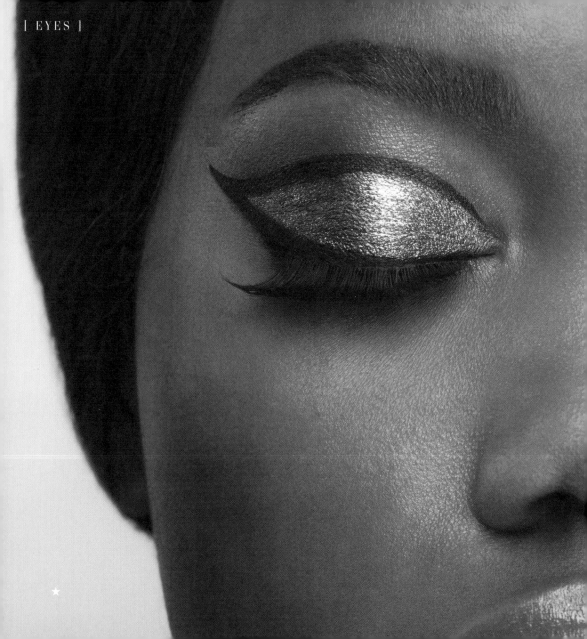

★

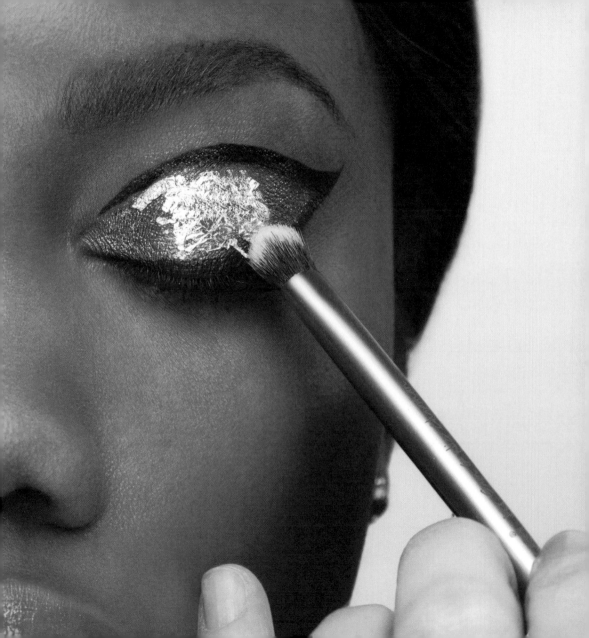

## USING EMBELLISHMENTS

Sequins and gold leaf are probably not something you would use every day but they add something different for a special occasion or creating a look for an editorial or fashion week.

## GOLD LEAF

Gold leaf is super-fiddly and fragile but it gives an amazing finish. It's available in a book of fine golden sheets or already cut into pieces in a pot, as well as in different colours.

Gold leaf adheres to the skin but it's best to use a cream eyeshadow as a base. You can still apply powder eyeshadow on top of the cream.

After applying the rest of your make-up, simply cut the gold leaf to the desired shape or tear it into handy pieces. Using a pair of tweezers, place the leaf onto the lid and, with a firm brush, press it down onto the skin. Brush off the excess with a soft, fluffy brush.

## SEQUINS AND GEMS

Online specialist make-up stores have a good variety but we often just pop down to our local craft shop and pick them up for half the price.

Dot a small amount of regular eyelash glue onto the back of the gem or sequin and tweeze it onto the skin. Apply a small amount of pressure for a few seconds to secure the gem.

To take off, use an oily eye make-up remover and gently pat over the area. After a few seconds it will lift off.

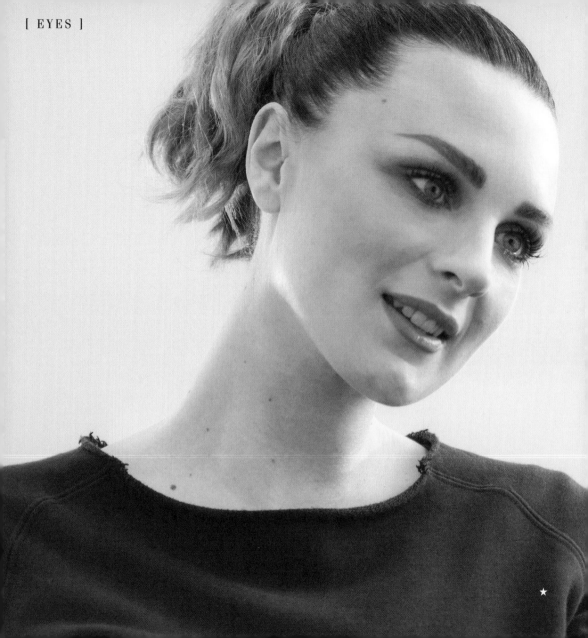

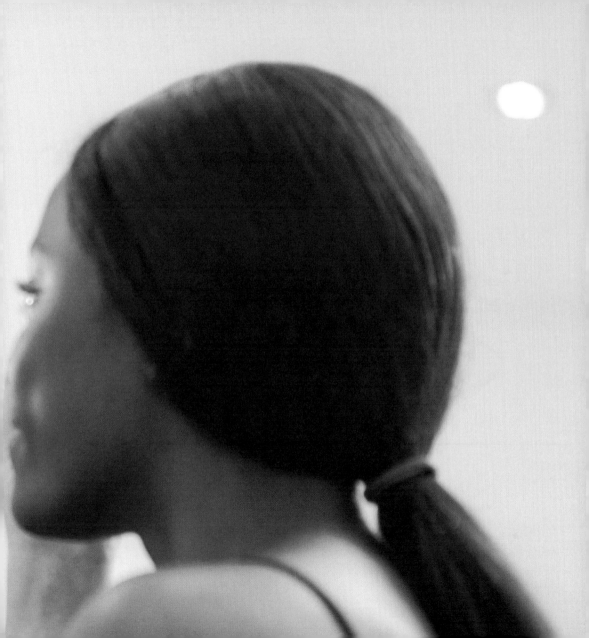

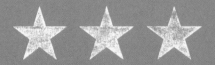

# *PIXI TIPS*

## [ EYES ]

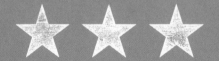

**1**

To avoid eyeshadow drop-down staining your cheeks we recommend Shadow Shields – paper segments that adhere to the under eye and project out to catch fall-out. You can purchase these online.

**2**

Cotton buds (or Q-tips) are a must-have for all beginners in make-up. Choose buds with one pointed tip and one paddle-shaped tip. The pointed end gets really close to the eye and under the lashes to clean up mistakes. The paddle end evens patchy areas of make-up and blends when you are on the go.

**3**

Loose-powder eyeshadows can also be used as blushers. Use sparingly as they are often strongly pigmented.

**4**

Glitter is notoriously hard to remove from your skin (and carpet and bed linen!). Our favourite tool to pick up ultra-fine glitter is micropore tape and an orange stick (a fine, wooden stick with one angled and one pointed end). Alternatively, you could use a brush handle. Wrap a piece of the micropore tape around the stick, sticky side out. Roll the stick along the skin and under the eye.

**5**

Buff a small amount of your concealer around the edge of the finished eye using a fluffy brush. This helps correct uneven eyeshadow shape and brightens the edge of your eye make-up.

# LASHES

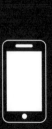
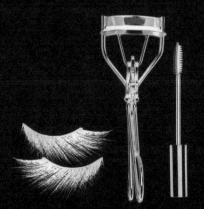

*"At sixteen, I was a funny, skinny little thing, all eyelashes and legs. And then, suddenly people told me it was gorgeous. I thought they had gone mad."*

———————————— *Twiggy*

*CORRECTLY* APPLIED *MASCARA ENHANCES* THE *APPEARANCE* OF *YOUR LASHES* AND *TRANSFORMS* THE *SHAPE* OF THE *EYE*.

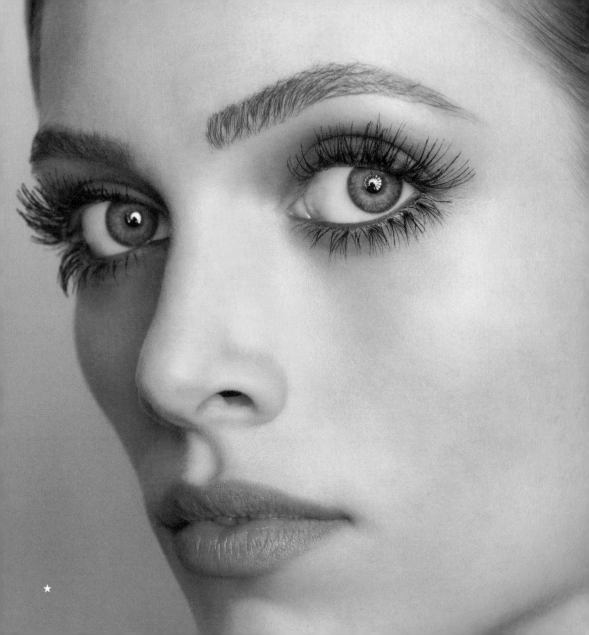

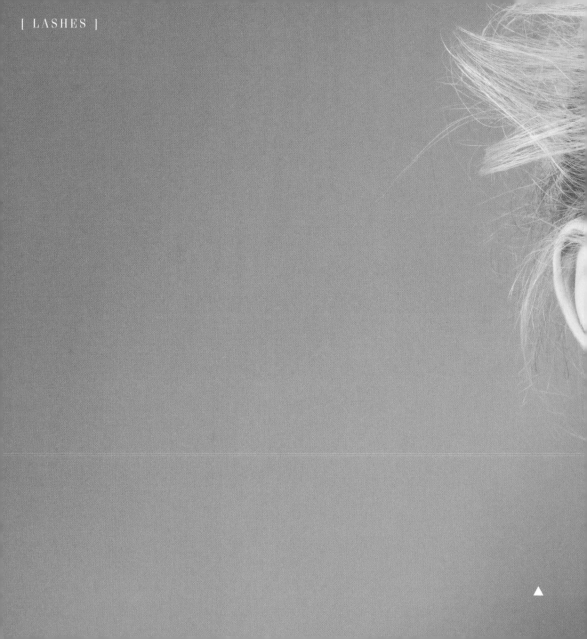

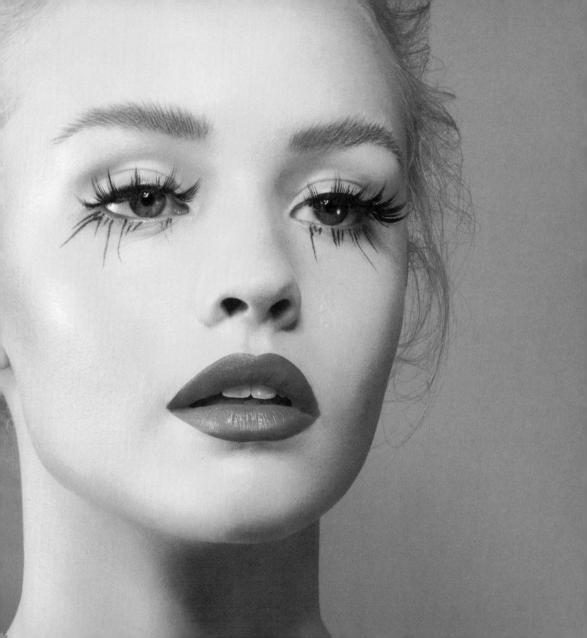

*YOU'RE PROBABLY WONDERING WHY LASHES HAVE THEIR OWN SECTION! BUT FOR SUCH A TINY PART OF THE FACE, THEY HAVE A HUGE IMPACT ON YOUR MAKE-UP AND HOW YOU FEEL AROUND OTHERS.*

THEY PROTECT THE EYE FROM DUST AND OTHER FLOATING PARTICLES, AND OVER THE YEARS WE HAVE BEEN ENHANCING THEM TO COMPLEMENT OUR IMAGE. CORRECTLY APPLIED MASCARA ENHANCES THE APPEARANCE OF YOUR LASHES AND TRANSFORMS THE SHAPE OF THE EYE.

For those of us who aren't blessed with naturally long, thick lashes there are numerous products to help. The life cycle of lashes ranges from 60 to 120 days and it can feel like an age before they regrow. Lash treatments are more popular for that reason and here we'll look at the best methods for managing your lashes.

## [ LASH TREATMENTS ]

### LASH PERMING

Lash perming is less popular these days, but it's good for people who have very short or dead straight lashes and is not as laborious as getting your hair permed. It doesn't require the same harsh chemicals, but you will be lying still for 20 minutes with your eyes shut while someone fiddles about with your lashes, so it's not ideal for the claustrophobic or anxious.

A tiny roller coated in adhesive is placed at the tips of the lashes and rolled backwards to the base. A solution is applied which helps hold the curl and is removed after about 20 minutes.

The curl can look a little too extreme but it drops after a few days and you are left with nicely curled lashes without needing mascara.

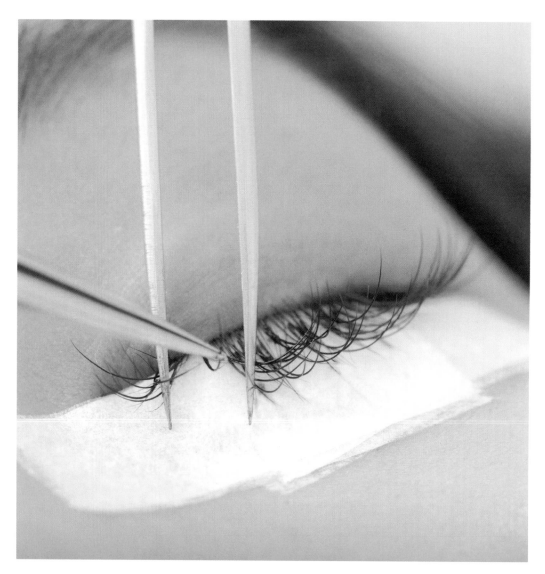

## LASH EXTENSIONS

Please do your research on this treatment. There are some seriously dodgy salons out there. Get recommendations from friends, research online and always go for a consultation before committing. Ask for images of their work and discuss the options available.

Extensions are usually either synthetic, silk or mink. Please do check how the mink hair is sourced at your consultation. A good salon will know the answer. Lashes range from natural and corner only to medium and long, as well as bottom lashes. Always go one length shorter as they'll look more extreme than you think they will. Add just a few for volume or go for a full set.

False lash hairs are tiny and resemble your natural lashes. A specialist adhesive is applied to one of your natural hairs and the extension is gently applied on top (see page 108). This treatment is very tedious, taking up to two hours and often salons charge you both for the treatment and then for the time on top.

Well-applied lash extensions start to drop out after about four weeks and will last around six weeks unless you have them in-filled so they don't look gappy and uneven. Occasionally, when the extension falls out it will take your natural lash with it.

# LASH *TINTING IS GREAT* IF YOU *HAVE SPARSE* OR *FAIR LASHES.*

Extensions offer you temporary volume and length and are perfect for a special occasion. However, make-up artists often dislike them because you can't apply mascara as its oil weakens the bonding glue and makes the lashes fall out.

## LASH TINTING

Our favourite treatment and something we do regularly ourselves. Lash tinting is great if you have sparse or fair lashes, can't be bothered to wear mascara every day or will be swimming on holiday.

If you are heading to a salon rather than doing it yourself, ensure they do a patch test 24 hours before your treatment. The therapist will apply a small amount of dye to an inconspicuous area – for example, behind the ear – to ensure you don't have an allergic reaction to the tint.

Tints are available in varying shades of brown and black. The darkest colour is usually blue/black.

The tint and a solution are mixed together and applied to the lashes and is removed after around 15 minutes. Your natural lashes are a beautiful dark tone that defines the eyes without the use of mascara. This should last four to six weeks and doesn't harm your natural lashes.

## LASH GROWTH SERUMS

Serums are a clear fluid applied with a fine brush. It usually contains lots of nourishing and moisturising ingredients to help strengthen and thicken your existing lashes. Though it feels like you lose lashes in the beginning, they soon grow back and seem to be much longer. We used a product called LiLash (RapidLash is also meant to be effective). Be aware, though, these are quite pricey.

We have both tried and liked humble castor oil – it's cheaper too. Available from most pharmacies, the oil is rich in omega oils, fatty acids and packed with vitamin E. It is also antibacterial and antifungal.

Apply serums by coating the base of the clean lashes in the evening. If you apply it in the morning you may find you get an oily film over the eye. Mascara doesn't sit too well on top as it separates the product.

Apply castor oil using an old mascara tube, first giving it a good clean out. Don't forget to also clean the brush. Fill the tube with the castor oil and apply to the lashes using the wand. Go over your lashes with eye make-up remover in the morning before you apply your mascara.

*MASCARA* DOESN'T SIT TOO WELL ON TOP OF LASH GROWTH SERUMS AS IT *SEPARATES* THE PRODUCT.

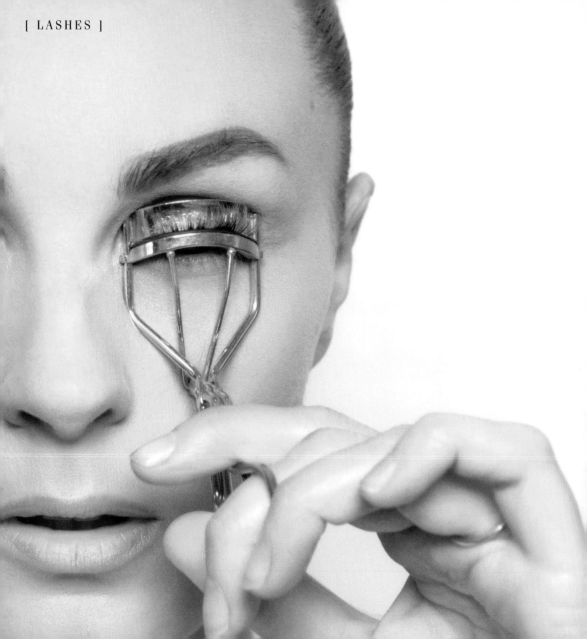

## LASH CURLERS

Lash curlers are the manual plastic or metal curlers used to curl your own lashes before mascara application. They may look like an implement for torture but they are effective and are something everyone should own because they make such a difference to shape. They instantly open the eye.

Curlers are available to fit different eye contours. The generic style is a softly curved metal clamp.

If you have hooded, small, deep-set or monolid eyes (see different eye types in 'Eyes', pp.28–47) you may prefer half-curlers. These are half the width of standard curlers and allow you to get closer to the root without nipping your skin. Clamp onto the lashes in three or four sections.

Lash curlers come with a thin rubber segment that sits inside the clamp, providing a cushioned base for the lashes. Some have a squared edge but we prefer those with a smooth, rounded edge to give lashes a softer, more natural curve. Replace the insert every three to six months as they wear and crack.

Keep curlers clean and dry to avoid damage or bacteria.

Ensure your hands are dry – we have seen people slip and pull lashes out with a wet hand.

We like to curl our lashes as we start our make-up, just after we apply skincare. It makes life easier: if you apply your eyeshadow first you may then disturb the powder and if you catch your skin and your eye waters you will ruin your base.

Heated lash curlers are good for people who are a little scared of the traditional clamp. Heated curlers look like a long wand that you hold against the lashes and brush up to gently bend the lashes back. The heat aids the curl and holds it in place.

After curling, apply your mascara as normal.

## FALSE LASHES

We love false lashes (or falsies), frequently using them in tutorials and wearing them on nights out. These days we are spoilt for choice with the different lengths, shapes, thicknesses, materials and textures available. Before you start, though, please make sure you read our section on applying false lashes (see p.120).

## STRIP LASHES

These cover the width of the whole eye and are secured onto a thin band. Strip lashes are made to fit all eye shapes, so you will probably need to trim them – start from the outer corner, where the lashes are the longest so you don't alter the natural gradient.

Good-quality strip lashes are usually made from real or mink hair, look soft on the eye, curve in a natural shape and blend with your natural lashes. Check that mink hair is sourced ethically. Synthetic lashes usually have a harder texture with a shiny finish.

Look closely at lashes before you buy them. Natural lashes should have finer hairs and be evenly spaced. Some have hairs that are longer or bunched together in certain areas, where they will draw attention. Consider your eye shape when deciding where the lash emphasis should be. Always go more natural than you think you want. False lashes look longer and more dramatic on the eye than in the packet.

You apply adhesive to the band, the strip from which the hairs protrude. The band's thickness depends on the length and weight of hair. Thicker bands are less flexible and are harder to apply and feel more uncomfortable. A natural band is more comfortable and also blends into the lash line easily.

## INDIVIDUAL LASHES

These look like an individual hair attached to a root bulb. Often there are three or four hairs attached to one bulb. You will usually get a row of short, medium and long lashes. In our experience, the long ones are best kept for creating an avant-garde look.

Apply adhesive to the bulb and slot between your natural lashes to fill gaps and create volume where needed. They are quite fiddly but give the best finish if you prefer a natural look. Shorter lashes are good anywhere, including on the bottom lash line, but keep medium and longer lashes for the outer corners.

We advise all our brides to wear this style of lashes on their wedding day. They feel comfortable, look great and are totally undetectable – if the bride cries and one falls off it's not the end of the world.

## CORNER LASHES

These are half or three-quarters of the length of standard strip lashes. The inner lashes are medium length and gradually lengthen to the outer edge. They give a feline look and create length at the eye's edge.

They feel comfortable on the eye and look beautiful with a flick of black liquid liner. Position these towards the outer corner of the eye and ensure you apply lots of mascara to the centre of the eye to blend in your natural lashes.

## LASH ADHESIVE

Some lashes have a sticky band and are ready to be applied straight away, while others are sold with lash glue.

This tends to get thick and gloopy so we advise buying a separate tube of lash adhesive. We love Duo, which has an easily controlled texture and dries clear.

It won't show up any little mistakes. It also comes in a darker colour and in a latex-free option.

## APPLYING FALSE LASHES

We prefer to apply our mascara before our lashes to make sure we don't pull at the false lashes later and dislodge them.

In addition, once you have applied your false lashes you can't reach the natural roots so easily. Avoid mascara on false lashes, which looks more obviously fake and synthetic, unless it helps with blending. Follow our steps and images:

# 1

Apply a small blob of glue to the back
of your cleansed hand.

# 2

Gently drag the band of the lash through the glue.

# 3

Ensure the band has an even but thin covering.

# 4

Wave the lash for around 30 seconds so that the glue dries slightly to stop it slipping and sliding over your eyelid or sticking your lashes together.

# 5

Looking down into a mirror, position the centre of your lashes and push each corner down.

# 6

The lashes should sit on the skin at the point where your natural lashes project. Adjust them slightly if needed and then push them in sections into the skin.

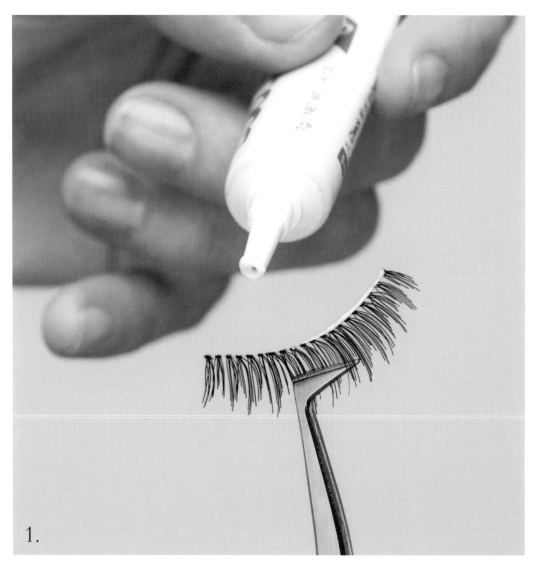

1.

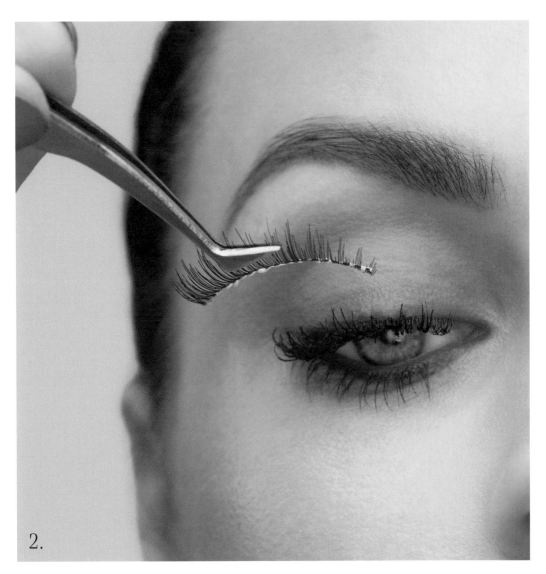

2.

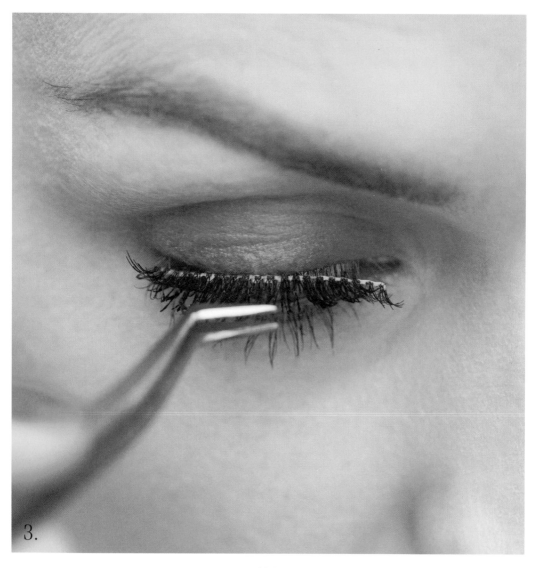

3.

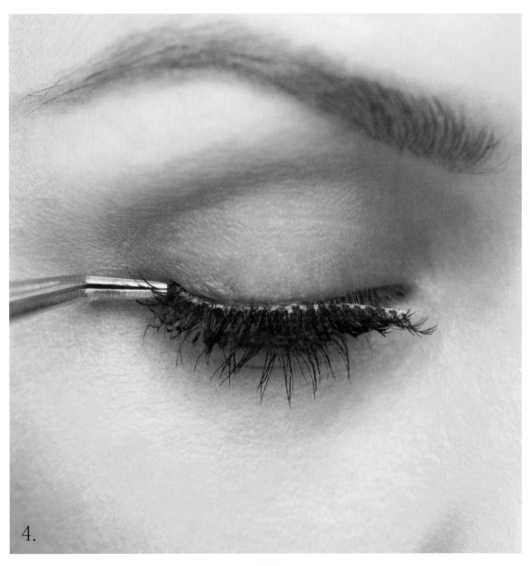

4.

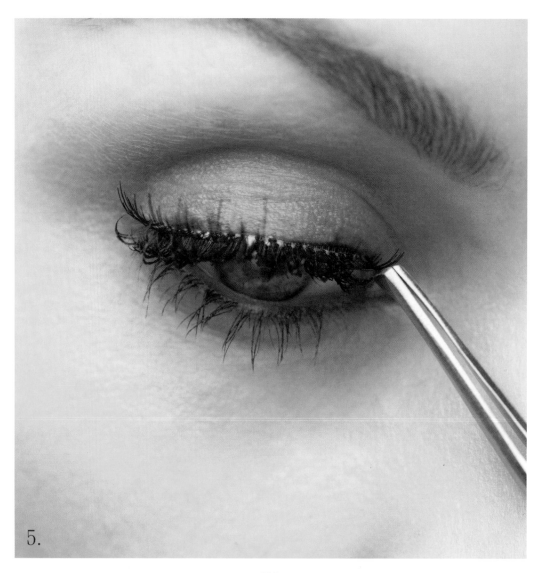

5.

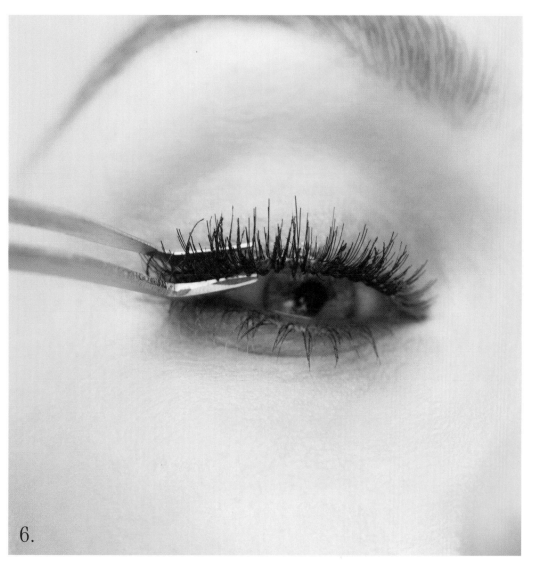

6.

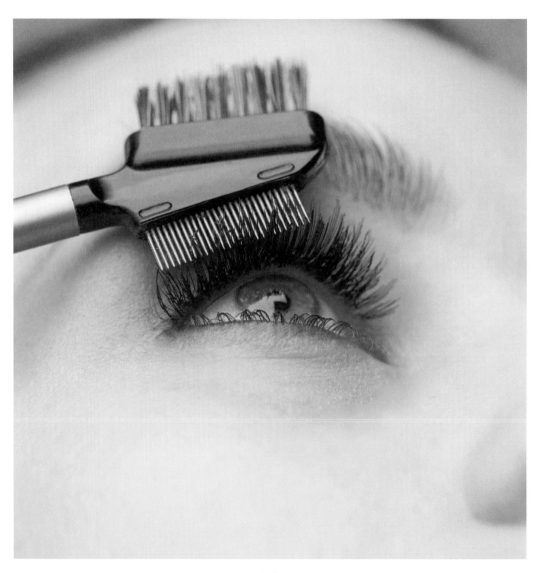

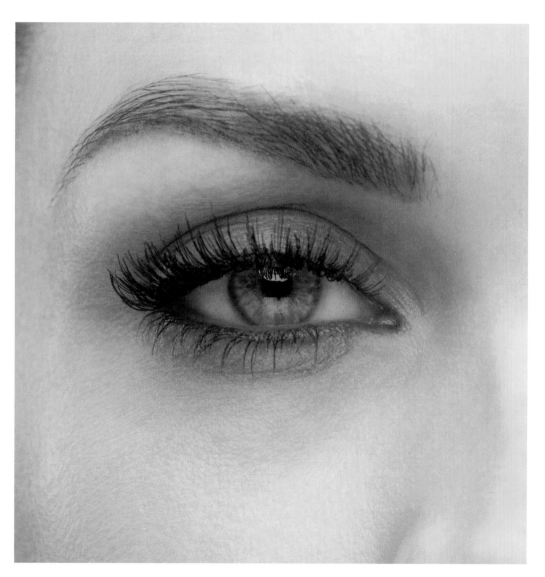

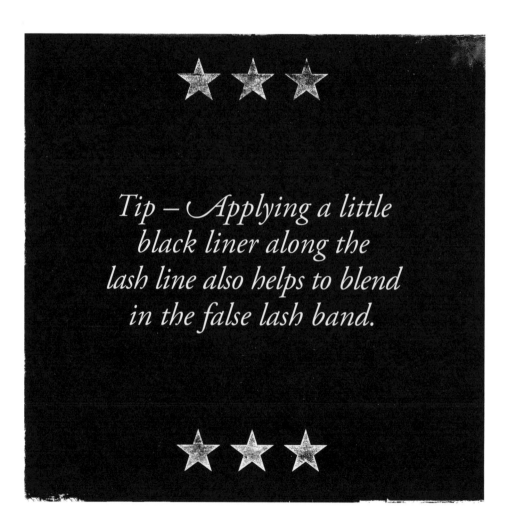

*Tip – Applying a little black liner along the lash line also helps to blend in the false lash band.*

## REMOVING FALSE LASHES

# 1

To remove, first saturate a cotton pad with an oil-based
eye make-up remover.

# 2

Hold the pad over the base of the lashes for a few seconds
and then gently pull the lashes away from the skin.

# 3

Clean any residue off the falsies and pick away the dried glue.

# 4

You can usually use a pair three times before they start
to lose their shape.

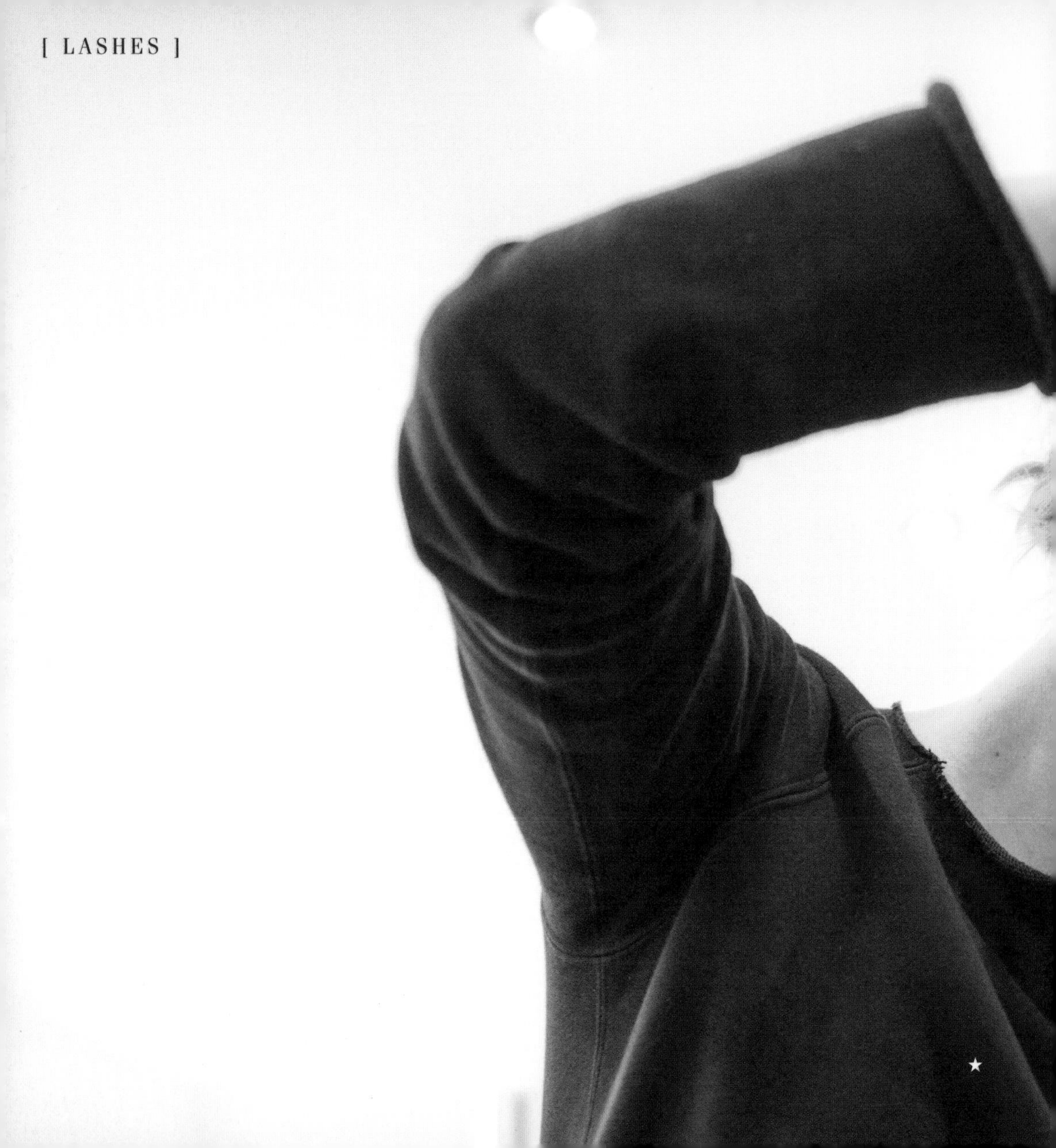

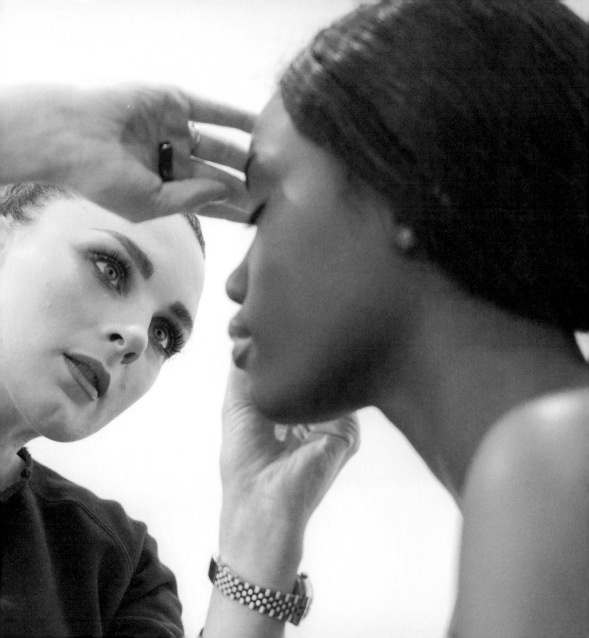

WE *LOVE FALSE LASHES (OR FALSIES)*, FREQUENTLY USING THEM *IN TUTORIALS* AND *WEARING THEM* ON *NIGHTS OUT*.

## LASH PRIMER

We don't bother too much with lash primer as it can make lashes look quite spikey and we prefer a softer-looking finish. Generally, it's good for sparse lashes, helping to create spidery lashes without needing to use as much mascara. Primers are white, black or clear and applied as you would mascara. Use primer to move and shape your lashes. It gives good separation.

## MASCARA

Anyone can wear mascara without needing tools or being overly skilled. It takes no time to apply and is an instant pick-me-up.

Some brands seem to launch what they claim is a new, innovative mascara every month but, to be honest, while brushes and a few ingredients change they are all pretty similar. Different brush heads suit different eye shapes and growth of lashes:

### SYNTHETIC MASCARA WANDS

These have plastic-looking brush heads. The bristles look quite spikey, feel firm and are slightly less flexible. The brush is usually slim. Good for people who need definition and lash separation and have fine, short or sparse lashes.

### COMPACT, NATURAL BRISTLE WANDS

These have lots of fine bristles tightly packed onto the wand and are usually chunky and large. The larger barrel of the brush means the lashes curl around and have a greater bend, looking less defined but much fuller.

Product transfers easily, making it difficult to apply to smaller, close-set or hooded eyes. Good for long lashes and large eyes.

### TAPERED WANDS

These have a triangle-shaped brush head ending in a small point. Greater space between bristles means more definition and volume. The tapered point catches fine lashes at the inner corner of the eyes and the bottom lashes. Use the end of the wand to pick these individual hairs out.

### BOTTOM LASH MASCARA

These mini-brushes are also super-slim so that you can coat the bottom lashes with ease without product transfer. They take forever to achieve a good coating on top lashes.

### FIBRE MASCARA

Tiny nylon fibres, applied via the brush wand, act like extensions by clinging to the lashes and create length and volume. They drop easily if you rub your eye and we don't advise using them if you have sensitive eyes or contact lenses.

*ANYONE* CAN *WEAR MASCARA WITHOUT* NEEDING *TOOLS* OR BEING *OVERLY SKILLED.* IT TAKES *NO TIME* TO *APPLY* AND IS *AN INSTANT PICK-ME-UP.*

## WATERPROOF MASCARA

This comes with all styles of brush head but we don't often wear it because it's such a pain to remove. Good for watery eyes, living in a humid country or if you are likely to cry.

## COLOURED MASCARA

Popular back in the 1980s, it's making a comeback. Everyone's mum (and maybe dad) owned an electric blue mascara! We can thank Debbie Harry and Princess Diana for that. It can really enhance the eyes and doesn't always have to look dramatic.

You can apply from root to tip of the lash, but for a subtle finish try adding a complementary colour to the tips. We enjoy wearing coloured mascara on the bottom lashes in a vibrant colour during the summer to add something special to a natural look.

Apply straight onto bare lashes or on top of a black mascara to soften the look. For intense, vibrant lashes, paint on a white mascara, leave to dry and then cover with colour.

## LASH LOSS

Lashes naturally fall out and then regrow (usually in a six-to-eight week cycle), although certain medication, disorders or alopecia can also induce loss. If your lash loss is a result of medication, stay positive and know that they will grow back, usually longer and thicker than ever!

Certain types of alopecia mean that they will not grow any longer but there are ways to create an illusion of lashes.

Smudge a soft kohl pencil along the lash line in the colour of your choice to define the eyes and give the impression of lash darkness. Keep strip lashes fine and light to be natural.

Individual lashes work particularly well on the lower lash line. Use your kohl pencil to tight line the upper waterline by applying kohl to the fleshy part of the eye where the lashes project from on the upper lid (see liner section on page 86-91).

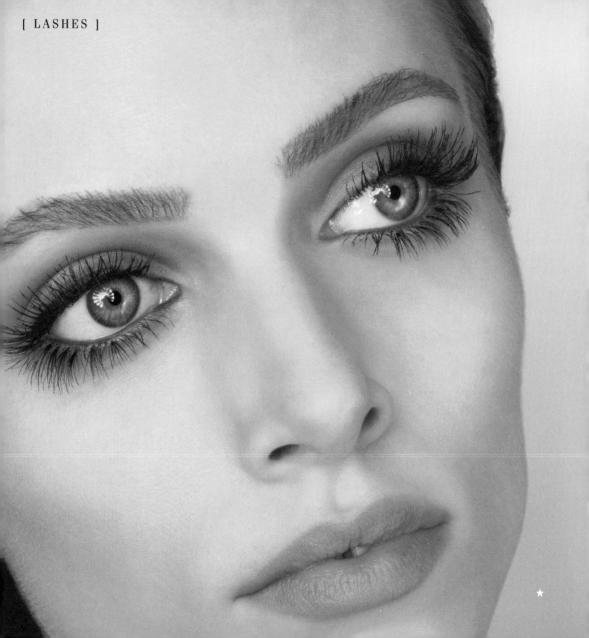

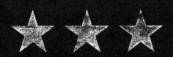

*Tip – Individual lashes
work particularly well on
the lower lash line.*

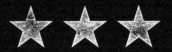

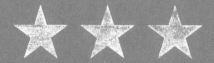

# PIXI TIPS

[ LASHES ]

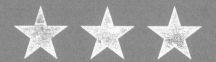

**1** Don't pump your mascara wand in the tube. It pushes in both bacteria and air, and can cause mascara to dry out.

**5** Plum-coloured mascaras enhance green and blue eyes. Green or blue mascara looks amazing on brown eyes.

**2** For extremely fair or red eyelashes, use a fine liner brush dipped into your mascara to paint product at the roots of lashes.

**6** Use an oil-based remover to take off waterproof mascara. It breaks down the product to make removal easier.

**3** Always follow the use-by date on your mascara to avoid eye infections.

**7** Always use a disposable mascara wand when working on others. Use a fresh wand for each eye and never double dip; you'll contaminate the product if your model has any eye infections.

**4** Brush your lashes through with a lash comb after applying mascara to reduce clogging and help to separate the lashes.

**8** Mascara on top of false lashes can look overdone. Apply mascara to individual lashes before sticking them down to avoid pulling them off.

# BROWS

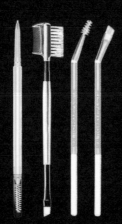

*"You must never underestimate
the power of the eyebrow."*

——————————— *Jack Black*

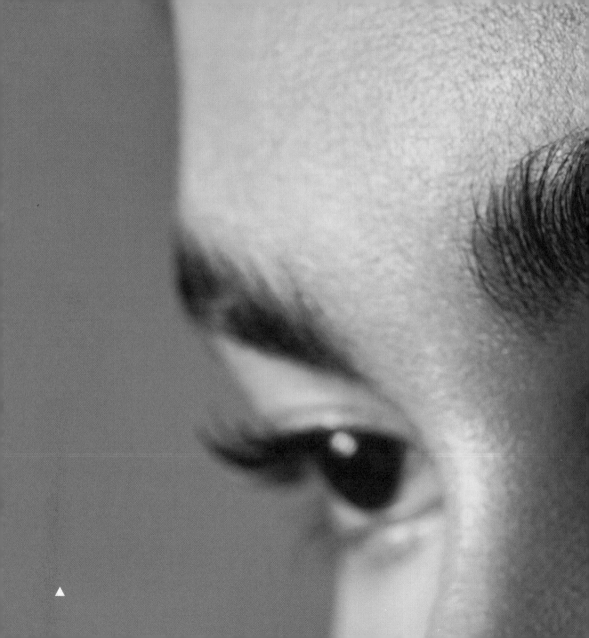

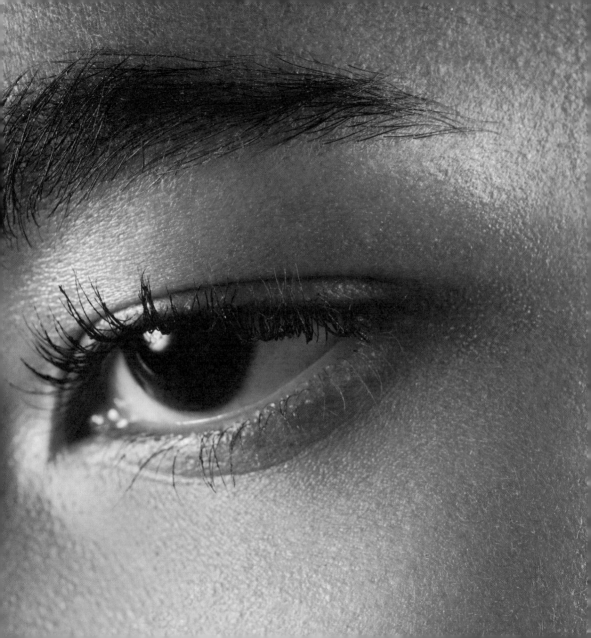

A *MINIMAL* AMOUNT
OF MAKE-UP *ON THE BROW*
CAN *MAKE* THE *BIGGEST*
*DIFFERENCE*, BUT
IT *CAN BE DIFFICULT*
TO *GET RIGHT*.

*BROWS HAVE BECOME THE BIGGEST TREND IN MAKE-UP AND BROW-SCULPTING IS ONE OF OUR MOST REQUESTED YOUTUBE TUTORIALS.*

A MINIMAL AMOUNT OF MAKE-UP ON THE BROW CAN MAKE THE BIGGEST DIFFERENCE, BUT IT CAN BE DIFFICULT TO GET RIGHT. COLOUR CHOICE MAKES A HUGE DIFFERENCE ALTHOUGH IT CAN BE TRICKY TO GET BROWS EVEN.

REMEMBER THOUGH, BROWS SHOULD BE SISTERS, NOT TWINS! MAKING THEM TOO SYMMETRICAL CAN LEAVE YOU LOOKING STRANGE.

## BROW SHAPES

A good brow should complement your eye shape and blend with your hair colour. First work out where your brow should begin and end:

Hold your brush vertically so it sits at the edge of the nostril and passes through the inner corner of the eye in a straight line. This shows where your brow should begin.

Hold your brush at the edge of your nostril and angle it so that it passes through the pupil of your eye. This is the highest part of your brow arch.

To see where your brow should finish, hold the brush at the corner of the nostril and allow it to pass along the outer corner of the eye. You can apply little brow pencil dots at each of these three points to help you as you use product.

This is also a good guide to follow when shaping your brows using hair-removal methods such as tweezing. Pluck the fine hairs that fall outside the area where you hold up your brush. There really are no rules when deciding how full to wear your brows.

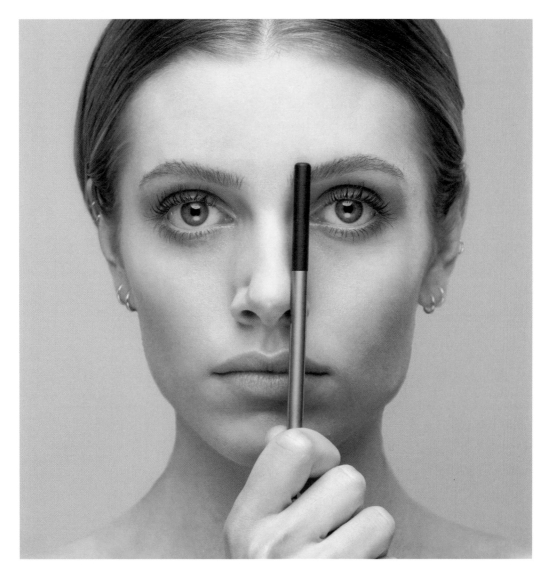

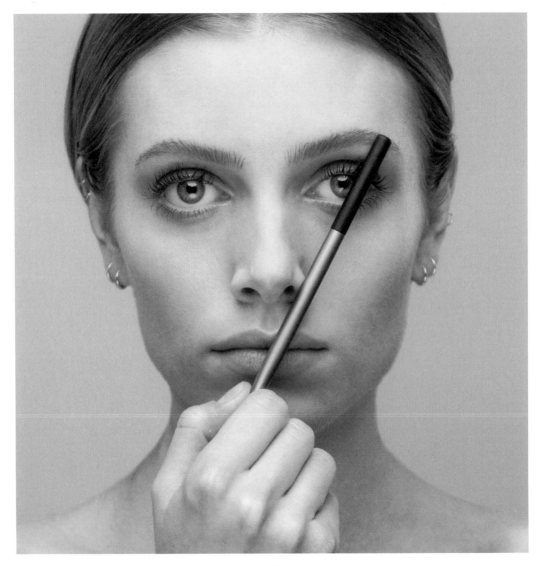

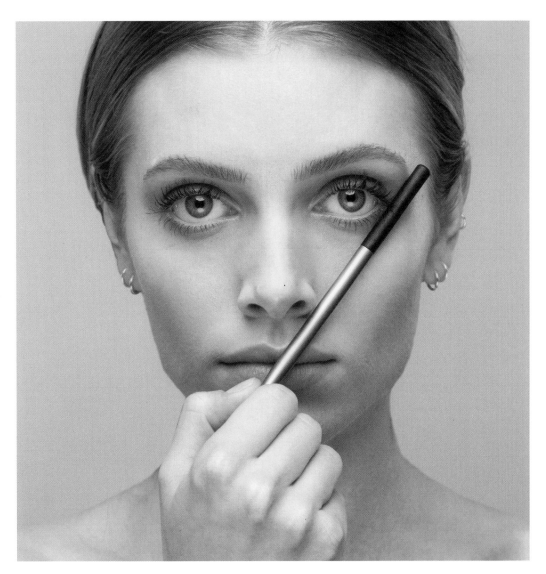

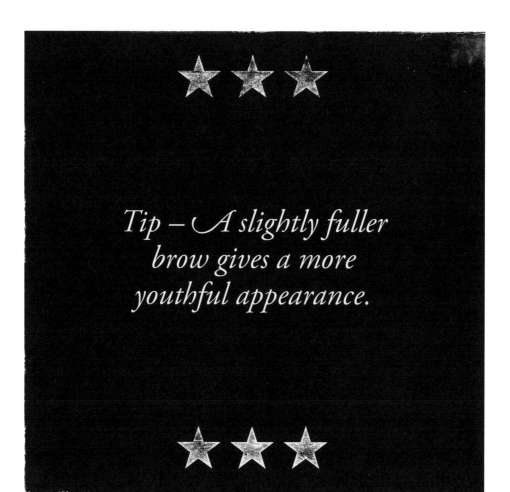

*Tip – A slightly fuller brow gives a more youthful appearance.*

## BROW HAIR REMOVAL

If you are a little nervous about shaping and removing hairs, then go to a reputable salon. Get recommendations from friends whose brows you like or stop someone in the street and ask them where they go to get an immaculate brow shape. You'll make their day by asking!

If you have previously removed hair, wait around four weeks to ensure you or the therapist can grip onto the hairs easily. A good beauty therapist or brow specialist will always first ask:

What is your ideal shape? Do you have any images of brow shapes you like? How do your brow hairs fall? Are they fine or coarse hairs?

The therapist will take a close look at your brows before removing any hairs. The brow shape you have in your mind may not necessarily suit your face and a good therapist will be honest and advise you accordingly.

## TWEEZING

The most obvious hair-removal method is by using tweezers. Our favourite type is slightly angled, allowing you to rest them on the skin while getting close to the root. We find angled tweezers reduce the risk of nipping your skin.

Pointed tweezers are more difficult to use because they cover a smaller surface area. They can also be a little stabby. They are good for teasing out tiny stubbly hairs or ingrown hairs. Tweezers with a squared-off end grip hairs but nip easily.

Ensure you pull hair as close to the root as possible in the direction of hair growth to avoid causing the hair follicle shape to distort. Otherwise the next hair may grow at a weird angle or become ingrown.

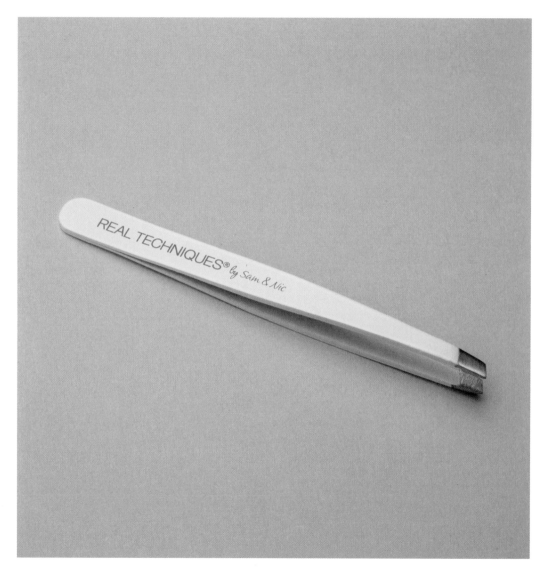

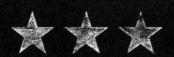

*Tip – Waxing is quicker
and less painful than tweezing
and regrowth is slower.*

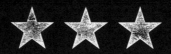

## WAXING

We wouldn't advise doing this yourself as you can't stretch the skin and remove the wax easily on your own.

Strip wax is applied to the skin in the direction of hair growth and removed using a cloth or paper strip in the opposite direction. Strip wax is softer and has a more gloopy texture. It can be used on the brow, but it's better on larger areas of the body.

Hot wax is thicker, dries quickly and sets hard onto the hairs rather than the skin. It is usually applied against the hair growth so that it pushes the hairs up before a second layer is applied.

It's left to dry off and harden before being pulled off against the direction of hair growth. Hot wax is effective on smaller areas of the body. It can be easily controlled and doesn't require cutting up cloth strips into tiny pieces.

## THREADING

Threading has been around for a long time in Asia but has become popular in the West over the last five years.

A fine piece of cotton thread is dragged along the skin in a twisting motion, trapping the hairs and pulling them out at the root. It not only removes the darker hairs but also the very fine, downy hairs that often show up under powder eyeshadow. Make-up sits beautifully on a threaded brow. It's very precise and effective on problem hairs or very coarse hair. Super-quick and no more painful than tweezing hairs, it's also great for sensitive skin that reacts to chemicals.

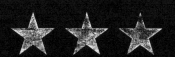

*Tip – Make-up sits
beautifully on
a threaded brow.*

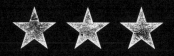

## ELECTROLYSIS

Electrolysis is not as popular as it once was. It's a long process that can be quite costly and must be performed by a qualified therapist.

A fine needle is inserted into the hair follicle through which an electrical current is passed into the root of the hair. The root is destroyed and the hair removed using tweezers. The hair should be growing and so requires regular treatments to ensure it's zapped at the optimum time.

## HD BROWS

You may have heard a lot of journalists and online gurus talking about HD Brows. We think this technique is responsible for the huge popularity of brow-shaping and probably guilty of encouraging people to become obsessive about their brow shape!

HD Brows is the brand name for a technique that basically combines all the approaches we have mentioned. An initial consultation is followed by tinting, waxing, threading, tweezing, trimming and after-care. Perfect for sculpted brows but if you prefer a more natural look we suggest sticking to your tweezers.

## BROW TINTING

You may have very fine brow hairs that don't require hair removal but need tinting to add volume. We often tint our own brows using a home-dye kit before plucking. It darkens the hairs, making them easier for us to see.

It's easy to purchase a kit and do it yourself. It creates volume, you no longer need to apply cosmetic brow products, it allows you to swim without fear of your brows moving and it tints your greying or white hairs.

Apply a barrier cream, such as Vaseline, around the brow to avoid the tint staining the skin. Mix your tint up according to the instructions and, using a disposable mascara wand, gently brush the tint through the brow hairs. You can apply a thicker layer depending on the intensity. The longer you leave the tint on, the darker the colour.

Brow tinting is especially effective on red hair or silver and greying hair. However, due to the coarseness of red or grey hair you may need to leave the tint on for longer.

## SEMI-PERMANENT BROW MAKE-UP

Having your brows tattooed on is the norm for some people and the number of salons offering this treatment are vast, so be sure to do your research. All good salons offer a consultation first.

The most natural semi-permanent brow is created using feathered hair strokes. It takes time and patience but in the end you will be left with a perfect brow that resembles natural hair.

A local anaesthetic is usually used to reduce sensitivity as the colour pigments are applied to the brow area using a fine needle.

This treatment will generally last from nine months to a year and a half depending on how your skin reacts with the pigment.

## BROW BLEACHING

If you have naturally dark brows, it's almost impossible to make them appear lighter using traditional eyebrow make-up products. You'll just end up with some weird tone that makes your brows even more obvious. We think light hair and darker brows looks fab but we have actually done this when we've lightened our hair and felt our brows were too dark. However, our brows are very sparse so it didn't look drastically different.

Please proceed with caution. Bleaching treatments need to be applied and left on the brow hair for not much longer than one minute. They take to the hair extremely quickly.

Some hairdressers offer brow bleaching but there are also lots of good brow-bleaching products – but never use normal household bleach. If your brows are naturally dark brown or black then we would advise getting this treatment done with a hairdresser as you run the risk of getting orange- or copper-coloured brows!

THERE ARE *TONS OF BROW PRODUCTS* AVAILABLE TO CREATE *DIFFERENT TEXTURES AND FINISHES.*

## BROW PRODUCTS

There are tons of brow products available to create different textures and finishes. For the most natural finish you need to use small amounts of a few different products.

### BROW PENCILS

Probably the most common type of brow product. Most brands will do brow pencils in a wide variety of shades. Pencils give a very defined one-dimensional finish to the brows and are good for filling in sparse areas or for creating shape.

Don't simply fill in your brows in a block colour. Use the pencil to create tiny, hair-like flicks. We like to use a disposable, clean mascara wand to brush through the pencil to soften the finish.

Quite often brow pencils also have a spooley-style brush to shape the hairs and soften the pencil. You should go for a pencil that feels harder and waxy. It will last longer on the skin, although it will require more pressure on application. A softer pencil will move in humidity and transfer easily.

## BROW CREAM

These are pigmented creams with a hard texture. By creating tiny, hair-like flicks, you can build shape and colour and creams also colour the skin underneath the brow. They create a more natural texture, rather than the block finish of a pencil. We like to apply brow cream products with a very fine synthetic angled brush. Use the point of the brush to create fine hairs and the angle of the brush to draw the shape.

## BROW GELS

Brow gels (p.171) look like a mascara but are specifically for the brows. Tinted brow gels brush through the hairs and provide colour. You can apply gels over any other brow product. They set the brows and give texture to the hair. They catch fair hairs too, making them stand out.

## BROW STAIN

Liquid brow colour applied using a felt-tip pen-style applicator. These provide a one-dimensional colour and must be used in small, hair-like strokes. These are also quick-drying – so work quickly or they will stain the skin. Brow staining is good in humidity and is long-lasting but needs practice.

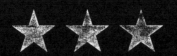

*Tip – Ensure your pencil
is always sharp so you can
get a precise finish.*

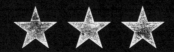

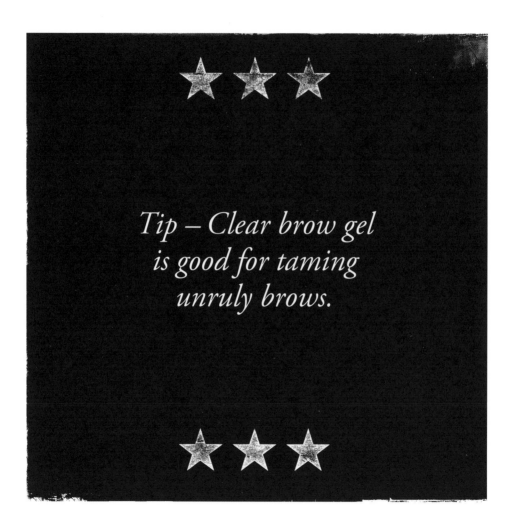

*Tip – Clear brow gel is good for taming unruly brows.*

## CHOOSING BROW COLOUR

The most important factor in achieving a beautiful, natural-looking brow. If you prefer a dramatic brow in a bold tone then feel free to skip this section!

If you have dark hair, go for a lighter colour than you think you need to ensure they blend in and don't look blocky. If you have light brows, you need to go for a similar colour to your own hair but in a cool, ashy tone. These also work well on red hair.

Brows are never just one colour and you may need to use two shades to create a natural finish. Use a slightly darker shade on the underside of the brow and through the front of the brow and use a similar shade to your natural hair through the main body and ends of the brow. Your brows are naturally darker in these areas, so continue with this depth of tone.

Our favourite brow brand is by Anastasia Beverly Hills. They have brow powders with a lighter colour and a darker colour in one pot to allow you to mix shades.

## BLONDE HAIR

Don't choose a colour that is too warm (by warm, we mean a shade with a golden or orange undertone). These don't blend and will look obvious. Go for an ashy tone with an almost greyish colour. You can always add some light strokes of an ashy brown.

It may feel alien to have any colour applied to very fair hairs, so you can use a slightly tinted, taupe brow gel. Gently brush the gel through and remove any excess with a clean brow brush.

## BRUNETTE HAIR

Possibly the easiest hair colour to match, but look closely at the undertones of the hair to establish the tone. Use a lighter tone than you think you will need. This way you can build the colour to add depth. If you have a lot of red tone you can add an auburn colour.

## RED HAIR

While red hair can be coarse – making brows look stiffer, thicker and even a little wavy – red brows can be extremely fair and almost non-existent.

If your hair is strawberry blonde then choose a similar tone with a caramel or honey tone. Ashy tones work really well.

For rich, auburn hair colour, go for a soft reddish-brown – almost chocolate. Your brows shouldn't be as dark or as bright as your hair colour.

## BLACK HAIR

If you are lucky enough to have jet-black hair then you can go either natural or extreme. If you are not confident in filling in, avoid using a pure black brow shade as you may end up looking like an evil Disney character. Always opt for a cool-toned black and avoid reddish undertones.

## GREY/SILVER HAIR

Grey hair can have a similar texture to red hair and can be quite wavy. Trim back unruly brows. A clear brow gel helps wavy hair to lay flat.

Facial features can become lost when the brow hairs turn white or silver but by applying a light taupe- or ash-coloured powder the eyes are framed and look stunning. A brow powder or pencil is best to ensure natural blending.

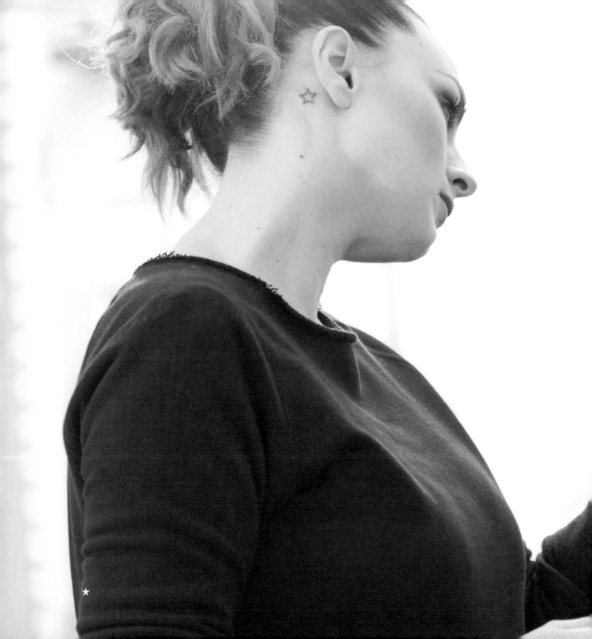

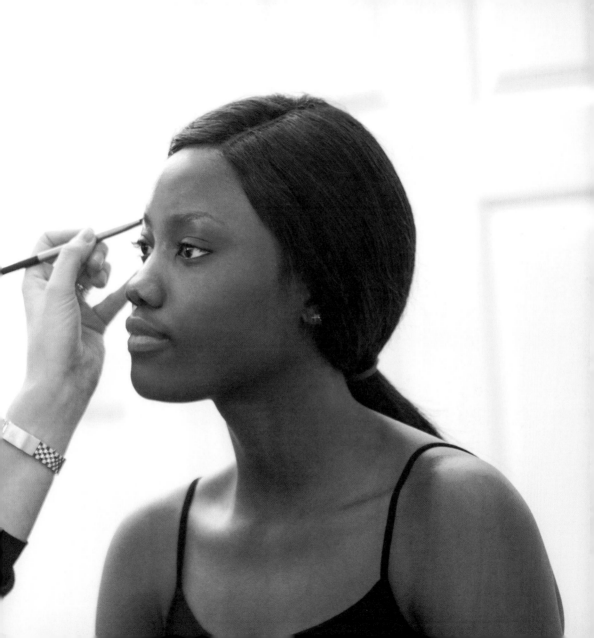

BE *GENTLE,*
USE *DELICATE*
*STROKES* AND TAKE
*YOUR TIME.*

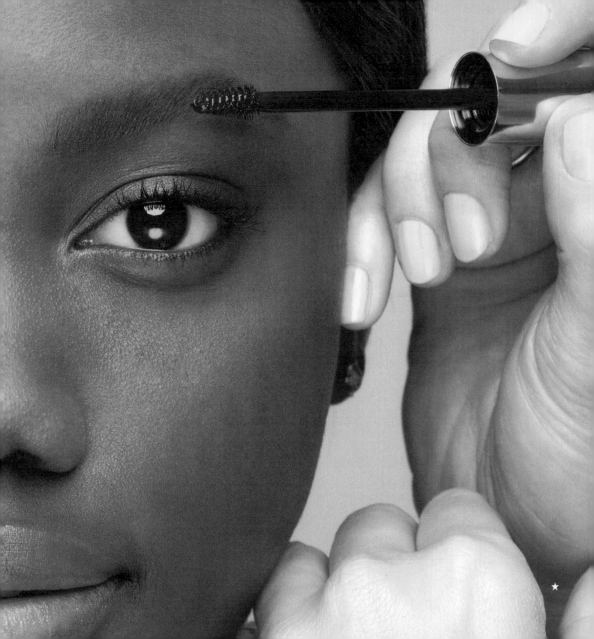

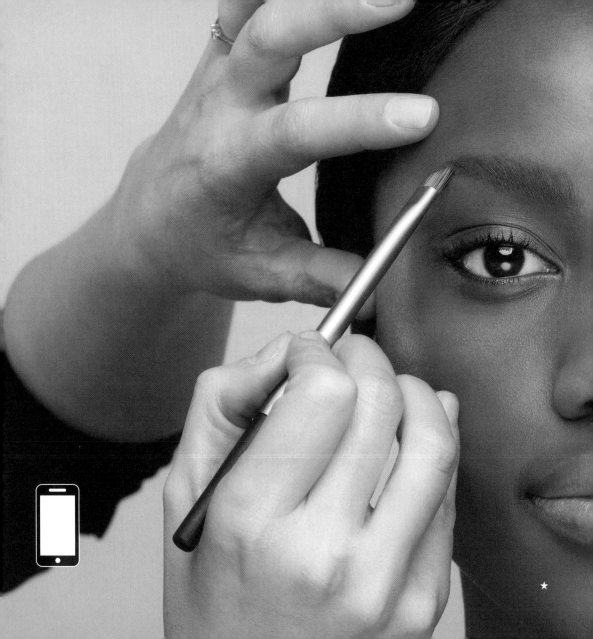

## APPLICATION TECHNIQUE

# 1

Be gentle, use delicate strokes and take your time. You can use a magnifying mirror on a stand. Just be sure to take a step back every so often.

# 2

Brush using a brow brush or spooley brush to see how the hairs lie and reveal the underside shape of the brow where you will be applying most colour.

# 3

In light strokes resembling hairs, begin to apply product to the front of the brow. Don't make this area too square.

# 4

Apply colour to the underside of the brow, working up to your arch.

# 5

Fill in the tail end of the brow. Avoid applying too much pencil to the top and thicken with soft strokes if necessary. Apply powder, cream or gel with a very fine angled brush.

We particularly like the Anastasia Beverly Hills No7 Brush. Brushes should be sharply angled and slim to recreate natural hairs. Use the shape of the angle to apply product in fine hair-like strokes. Use the point of the brush to apply product to the front.

# 6

Dampen your brush for more defined hair strokes. Once all products are applied, brush the brows to remove excess powder and to blend colours.

We like to finish our brows by brushing through a clear or slightly tinted brow gel. This sets the applied colour and also gives visible texture to the natural hairs.

# 7

For super-defined brows run a little concealer around the edge of the brow. Use a small shadow brush to apply the concealer close to the brow and using a fluffy brush, blend the concealer. It enhances the brow angles and takes down any skin redness.

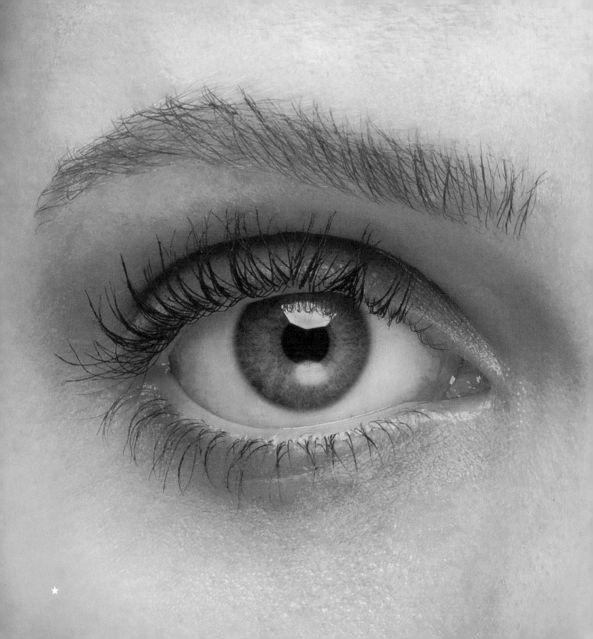

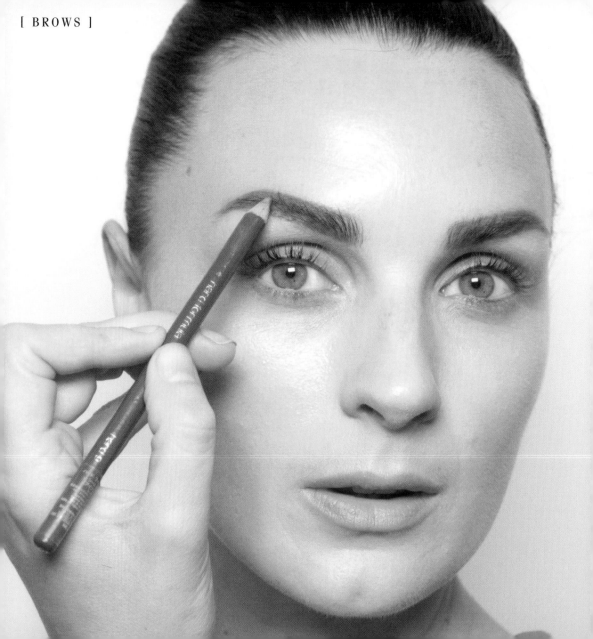

# FOR *FULLER* BROWS USE A *BROW* *GEL* TO *BRUSH* THE BROWS *UPWARDS*.

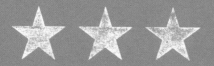

# *PIXI TIPS*

[ BROWS ]

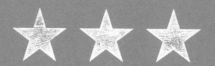

1

Brows are sisters, not twins. One brow often sits higher due to the muscle tone underneath. Don't try to make them too symmetrical.

2

One brow may have hairs sticking up or down. This is usually the side you sleep on. Try alternating the side you sleep on or invest in a silk pillowcase that won't grip the hairs.

3

Steam your face over a bowl of hot water or hold a warm face cloth on the brows for five minutes. This opens the follicles and allows hair to be plucked with a little less pain!

4

We all have those fine, downy hairs around the brow. These pick up fake tan or foundation that has been applied to the skin, giving you a weird orange fuzz around the brow. Avoid applying foundation over the brow and blend any overlap with a small fluffy brush.

5

Train unruly brows to sit in the direction of your choice. Before bedtime, give the brows a good brushing upwards and brush through some Vaseline or castor oil. This helps hairs to lie flat and over time they will begin to behave. Castor oil is also good at helping hair growth.

First, we would like to say a massive thank you to all of our followers, who have supported us on this crazy and exciting journey. Without you it wouldn't be possible. X

Thank you: Gleam Futures, our fantastic management. You're the best of the best; it's rare to find managers that really and truly have the best interests of their clients at heart. You look after us so well. Dom, Francesca, Abigail, Viv and all the rest of the team, it's an absolute honour and pleasure to have your help and get to work with you daily. (Also, Sam apologises if anyone is ever offended by the overuse of swearing in her emails.)

Thanks to Dundas Communications: Max, Amy, Freya, Callum and Nancy, for helping to steer us in the best direction. Just like Gleam, you are a rare find.

Thanks to Blink for all your help with this book.

Thanks to our family: Mum, Ian, Steff, Danny, Brian, Lily, Ollie, Harry and Edie for supporting, entertaining and helping us along the way. Your positive attitude when times get hard always pulls us through and your help managing and juggling the children has been paramount to our success.

Thank you to our friends James Lincoln (for taking photographs with zero direction) ★, Simon Songhurst ▲ and Elisabeth Hoff ♦ for all their stunning photographs, without which this book would be rather dull to look at.

Thanks to Danny and Steve at Type & Numbers for designing this book so beautifully.

Thanks to Stacey for helping us with this book and being the best friend anyone could ask for. May the Armchair Detectives live on forever!

Thank you to Amy for eating all the biscuits, chocolates, marshmallows, cake pops, macaroons and sweets that come with the daily Pixiwoo post, so that we don't have to. We'll pay for your dental bills when your teeth fall out!

Pixiwoe

After both finding careers in the make-up industry, sisters Nic and Sam joined together to create the Pixiwoo brand. Their highly successful YouTube make-up channel has over two million subscribers, each video generating hundreds of thousands of views. Sam and Nic are the faces of the famous Real Techniques brush collection. The brand has taken off in the US, the UK and around the world. Sam and Nic continue to grow as top artistic consultants, writing columns for national magazines and newspapers, appearing on major network television as beauty experts, and editing their own digital magazine. They continue to develop their Pixiwoo brand through their YouTube tutorials, as well as doing make-up courses from their studio.

Also available by Sam and Nic Chapman:

# PERFECT
# SKIN

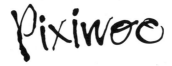

illustrated using original photography, this
beautiful compact book includes advice,
techniques and top tips on a variety of looks
and on how to work with your individual skin
tone and type for the best result.

Available from 5th October 2017
£9.99 RRP
ISBN: 978-1-911600-45-9

# PERFECT
# SKIN

## COMPACT MAKE-UP GUIDE

### TOOLS • SKIN • FINISHES

By the
REAL *by Sam & Nic*
TECHNIQUES®
artistic consultants

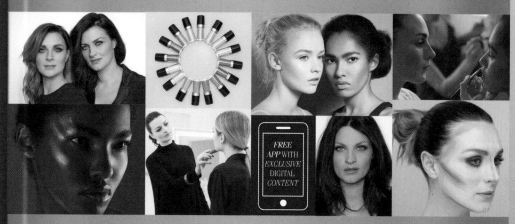

FREE
APP WITH
EXCLUSIVE
DIGITAL
CONTENT

*Pixiwoo*

SAM AND NIC CHAPMAN

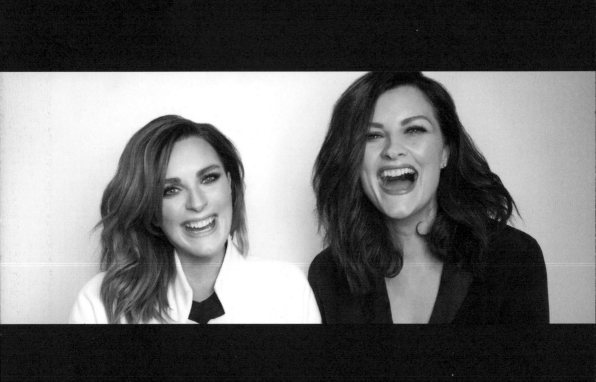